TWINS & MULTIPLE BIRTHS

*The essential parenting guide from
pregnancy to adulthood*

Dr Carol Cooper
in association with Tamba

Vermilion
LONDON

To my family, who are sometimes a challenge
but always an inspiration

9 10 8

First published in 1997 by Vermilion, an imprint of Ebury Publishing
This revised edition published by Vermilion in 2004

Ebury Publishing is a Random House Group company

Copyright text © Dr Carol Cooper 1997
Copyright illustration © Random House UK Ltd 1997

Dr Carol Cooper has asserted her right to be identified as the author of this Work in
accordance with the Copyright, Designs and Patents Act 1988.

The Random House Group Limited Reg. No. 954009

Addresses for companies within the Random House Group can be found at
www.rbooks.co.uk

A CIP catalogue record for this book is available from the British Library

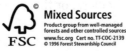

Mixed Sources
Product group from well-managed
forests and other controlled sources
www.fsc.org   Cert no. TT-COC-2139
© 1996 Forest Stewardship Council

The Random House Group Limited supports The Forest Stewardship
Council (FSC), the leading international forest certification organisation.
All our titles that are printed on Greenpeace approved FSC certified paper
carry the FSC logo. Our paper procurement policy can be found at
www.rbooks.co.uk/environment

Printed in the UK by CPI Mackays, Chatham ME5 8TD

ISBN 9780091894856

Copies are available at special rates for bulk orders. Contact the sales development
team on 020 7840 8487 or visit www.booksforpromotions.co.uk for more information.

To buy books by your favourite authors and register for offers, visit
www.rbooks.co.uk

This work cannot be exhaustive, and nothing in it is intended to be a substitute
for consultation with a medical practitioner or other professionals.

CONTENTS

ACKNOWLEDGEMENTS

I am greatly indebted to Tamba (the Twins & Multiple Births Association), who first agreed that there was a need for this book, and then entrusted me with the task of writing it. It would have been much less successful as well as less complete without the superb help of their honorary consultants, who have provided information and advice for both the first edition and this one.

I particularly want to mention Debbie Sen, Dr Helen Ball, Damian Eustace, Janet O'Keefe, Dr John Buckler, Jane Ellison, Peter Hendy-Ibbs, Rachel Hudson, Judi Linney, Pat Preedy, Audrey Sandbank, Gina Siddons, Jane Spillman, Jill Walton, Helen Forbes, Claire Edmonds, Diane Galloway and Carol Robins. I am also very grateful to Dr Elizabeth Bryan and Jane Denton at MBF (Multiple Births Foundation) for much expertise and support, Susanne Reid and the rest of the committee at IMBA (Irish Multiple Births Association), Professor David Hay and AMBA (Australian Multiple Births Association) who have allowed me to quote from the La Trobe Study, Professor Jim Stevenson, Dr Peter Tymms and Professor Jon Stallworthy. Naturally the comments and interpretation in this book are mine, and are not necessarily endorsed by Tamba or any other organisation.

Many twins, triplets and their families have been kind enough to let me repeat their spontaneous words and private thoughts. In all, a great many people have helped to stimulate my thinking and shaped this book. I hope I have not left anyone out.

Dr Carol Cooper, 2004

FOREWORD

I am delighted to see a second edition of this excellent book in print. When my twin girls were born in 1995 this valuable parenting guide was still at the manuscript stage and I was desperately scouring bookshops to get my hands on something practical and up-to-date that told it like it is.

Since the discovery of her own twin pregnancy, Dr Cooper has had a longstanding relationship with Tamba, the Twins & Multiple Births Association. Working together we have been able to combine a wealth of parents' experiences with current medical expertise and we are always particularly pleased to be involved with new literature relevant to parents and expectant parents of twins, triplets and more.

Much has changed in the seven years since this book was first published. The peak in multiple births that we saw in the 1990s appears to have evened out with fertility treatments being more closely regulated. However, the practical, emotional and financial implications of a multiple birth remain and the need for a book like this is still great. There is no getting away from the fact that multiple pregnancy is different and brings increased risks to the mother and babies. Many twins and nearly all triplets are born prematurely requiring additional care. Establishing feeding and sleeping routines can prove particularly difficult. Becoming a parent of two or more babies at once is a challenging experience for anyone but, with support and guidance, it can also be a very rewarding experience as the children grow up.

No one knows more than another parent what it is really like to bring up twins and Dr Carol Cooper is extremely well-qualified, as a GP and parent of teenage twins, to guide you in this role. This up-to-date book does not shy away from the realities of multiple pregnancy and parenting but is written in a very easy to read style. It is a comprehensive read written with authority and warmth. In particular, this new edition includes a revised section on breastfeeding and a whole new chapter on identity. *Twins & Multiple Births* is, most certainly, the essential parenting guide and will help parents meet the different challenges that twins or more can bring from day one through to adolescence.

Among the shelves of baby books and parenting manuals in the bookshops these days, this book should shine out to you as a parent of twins, triplets or more and to those of you still with time on your hands awaiting the babies' arrival!

Helen Forbes
Tamba Director, 2004

INTRODUCTION

To make sure you don't nod off, I must tell you now that this book is going to be about sex and money. Twins and higher multiples usually start off with sex, and always cost a lot of money.

When I was expecting my twins, I realised how much birth and parenting are geared towards having merely one baby at once. It was intensely frustrating to read about breast-feeding or bonding when no thought had been given to the fact that, for many mothers, their baby was planning to arrive in the world with at least one little pal in tow.

I found several excellent books on multiples, but some written from a parent's standpoint were getting out of date. I also wanted to include all the medical nuts and bolts that I know from experience people so often seek.

At the same time, my work as a family doctor made me conscious that the advice one so blithely dishes out may not be suitable for everyone. An author's ideal strategy can become a tyranny for others to follow. Society is hard enough as it is on imperfect parents and I feel strongly about some manuals which make readers feel deficient unless they do things in a certain way, or feel particular emotions for their children. We mums and dads don't have to be all-singing, all-dancing, and we can't all whip up gourmet meals like celebrity chefs either.

When you have twins, everyone around you is ecstatic. You're thrilled too. Or are you? If you don't already have children, you may not be over the moon at the prospect of an instant family and might have preferred to be broken in gently, like most parents. If you already have one child or more, you may find yourself even more short of arms and time. People admire twins, and strangers stop to chat but rarely offer help, and sometimes, worn out by the demands of intensive baby care, I would fleetingly envy mothers with singletons.

The reasons are simple. With twins, whatever one baby needs, the other may need too, and more or less at the same time! Twin pregnancies are more demanding physically and often mentally, and twin births of necessity have a higher rate of medical intervention. Because they are more likely to be premature or small, many babies born as multiples are admitted to the special care unit. Later, their parents face exhaustion from disruptive sleep patterns, the challenge of feeding two babies at once, the logistics of getting about, and the extra energy required in the rearing of more than one child at a time. Many mums and dads revel in these challenges, while others find solutions elusive.

I was fortunate to make contact early on with the Twins & Multiple Births Association (Tamba), which was founded in 1978 and supports families with multiples through local twins' clubs and specialist support groups. Since then, Tamba has gone from strength to strength and expanded its services, establishing The Freephone Twinline in 2003, its 25th birthday year. There are similar multiple birth organisations in other countries, and Tamba is a shining example to them.

When I was still pregnant, I also met Dr Elizabeth Bryan, who is widely regarded as the leading paediatrician in the care of multiples. My twins attended her first twins' clinic at Queen Charlotte's Hospital in January 1987, and the whole family has kept in close touch with her and the Multiple Births Foundation (MBF), which she launched in 1988. The MBF provides advice, information and support to multiple birth families and to all professionals concerned with their care. For professionals, there are MBF guidelines on a range of issues. GPs, health visitors, midwives and social workers can all approach the charity for information and advice, and parents can too.

Although very different, both Tamba and MBF play a part in promoting public and professional awareness of the needs of multiples. Tamba in particular campaigns on behalf of families. If my own experience is anything to go by, awareness is much needed because most of the population is unenlightened, and some can't even do simple arithmetic. One mother of four, who should have known better, asked me whether having twins was any different from having one baby. An otherwise intelligent friend said sceptically, 'If having twins or triplets is so hard, why do people always say how lucky you are?' Outside the school gates, another mother told me that having twins was so much easier than having one at a time. According to her logic, life with quads would have been a doddle.

As I learned more about multiples both from a practical point of view as a parent and from a medical angle as a GP, I realised that things could have worked out better for some parents of twins had they taken a different approach early on. With some juggling, parents can manage multiples, but what happens to the rest of the family? It takes skill and insight to balance the needs of twins with those of the other members of the household.

If you are feeling daunted, let me assure you that I have met many, many parents of twins and triplets (fewer with quads), and you are all special people. Better keep it to yourselves, lest friends who only have singletons feel inadequate, but you are élite mums and dads, the *crème de la crème*. As Premiership players, you take child-rearing to heights that the lower divisions can barely dream of. I know you are equal to the challenge.

The first edition of this book appeared in 1997, and has

been very successful. I am always honoured to hear how many paediatricians recommend it. I am especially grateful to the many special people everywhere who have told me that my book was their Bible and kept on the bedside table. But there is a lot going on in the world of multiples, and parenting books get dated a lot faster than bibles, so it is time for a new edition. This version takes in a lot of the new research findings as well as topics like baby massage that interest more and more parents.

When I spoke to audiences of Tamba members, at IMBA (Irish Multiple Births Association) and elsewhere, I realised how little information there was on adolescent and teenage twins. This is an area which parents find perplexing, to say the least, so that chapter is now far more detailed.

There is also a new chapter on identity and individuality, as these are issues that trouble twins and their families. We all want our children to grow up to become functional adults, but it's not easy when they arrive two at a time. Some parents, charmed by the notion of twins, may focus too much on the children's twin-ness, to the detriment of their development and sometimes of the other siblings' well-being too. Getting the balance right is part of the special mission for parents of multiples.

I have some of the answers, but – it may shock you to hear this from a medic – not all. Even if you are a first-time parent, you will have your own approach and will soon learn to trust your own instincts, not mine.

One final note: in common with many other childcare manuals, this book mostly follows the convention of female parent with male infants. This, of course, is done for the sake of clarity.

Chapter One

IN THE BEGINNING

Everything's different when you have twins. They're special, and the whole family becomes special too. It's like a virus everyone wants to catch.

The last twenty years or so have seen a huge upsurge in the numbers of twins, triplets and more, thanks to some of the social changes and medical advances explored later in this chapter. Since 1998, the rise in multiple births has been somewhat less dramatic, but even so there are more multiples born today than ever before. On average, there's now one set of twins for every 76 live births, making one baby in 38 a twin. In many developed countries, triplets and higher multiples are four to eight times more common than they were three decades ago. In 2001, 9,590 sets of twins were born in the UK. That same year, 235 sets of triplets also arrived, as did five sets of quads, one set of quintuplets and a set of sextuplets.

Even higher multiples can occur, but they're very rare. On 19 November 1997, Bobbi and Kenny McCaughey of Iowa, USA, became the first parents ever to deliver healthy septuplets. The arrival of the seven little superstars drew worldwide attention and more gifts than could possibly fit into their home. The highest recorded order is believed to be nonuplets, born to Mrs Geraldine Brodrick in Sydney, Australia, in June 1971. But her nine babies (four girls and five boys) survived only a few days.

Twins are perennially fascinating, and there have been many myths and misconceptions about them. According to beliefs held at various times, twins have been thought to represent good luck or fertility, to be infertile themselves, or, in the case of boy-girl pairs, to have indulged in incest in the womb. In medieval Europe, a woman bearing twins was often accused of adultery, and had to suffer the grim consequences.

Several mythological and religious figures have been twins, such as the Greek gods Castor and Pollux, the biblical pair Jacob and Esau, the Scandinavian gods Hoder and Balder, the Roman pair Romulus and Remus, who were raised by a she-wolf, and, in the Afro-Cuban religion Santería, the orishas who are the twin children of the god Chango and who fight and get up to all sorts of tricks. Famous twins include June and Jennifer Gibbons (the silent twins of Marjorie Wallace's book of the same name), Sir David and Sir Frederick Barclay, who are the wealthiest twins in Britain, and Ross and Norris McWhirter, who were able sportsmen as well as co-writers of *The Guinness Book of Records*. Many other twins have also found their twinship an advantage. Born in 1986, the Olsen twins, Ashley and Mary-Kate, have thriving careers as TV and film actors, and are now young business tycoons too. Dutch soccer legends Ronald and Frank de Boer, born in 1970, played for the same club for many years before separating to sign for Rangers (Ronald) and Galatasaray (Frank). In the world of cricket, there's the powerful duo Steve and Mark Waugh, and in the music industry famous twins include Luke and Matt Goss, formerly known as Bros. The best-known lone twin is probably Elvis Presley, but there is also Liberace, who was born Wladziu Valentino in Milwaukee, Wisconsin, in May 1919, weighing nearly 6 kg (13 lb), while his brother was stillborn. The singer Justin Timberlake is also a lone twin, his sister Laura having died at birth.

· *Types of Twins* ·

Am I a clone of him, or is he a clone of me?

Your own twins may never find fame or fortune, but they will be special. You can expect a huge amount of pleasure and fun, as well as a lot of attention wherever you go. As a parent of young twins, one of the first questions you'll be asked is, 'Are they identical?'

Pretty well everyone nowadays knows that there are two kinds of twin – identical and non-identical – though they don't always understand what causes the two types. And lots of mothers and fathers of twins aren't sure what kind they have.

So-called identical twins develop from the splitting of a single zygote or fertilised egg, and are more accurately referred to as monozygotic (MZ) or monovular twins. These twins almost always look very similar and can confuse those around them. In Germany, 19-year-old twins managed to escape a speeding fine because police didn't know who should face the charge: each of the women claimed the other one was driving at the time. One remand prisoner in the UK went on the run for nearly two years after changing clothes with his identical twin in a prison visiting room. However, both were eventually caught and jailed.

MZ twins are always the same sex, a fact which Shakespeare obviously failed to appreciate when he wrote the indistinguishable Viola and Sebastian into *Twelfth Night*, though since he had a boy-girl pair himself he should perhaps have realised it. MZ twins can only be of different sex if something goes slightly awry at the time of cleavage of the egg, so that one of the X chromosomes goes missing. This is extremely unusual, so to all intents and purposes MZ twins are always the same sex. They have exactly the same genetic material or DNA as each other. You could, if you like, consider them to be natural clones.

Non-identical twins are about twice as common as identical or MZ twins, and are no more alike (or dissimilar) in looks and personality than any other two siblings. They come from different sperms and separate eggs, in other words from two fertilised eggs (zygotes). Scientifically, it's more accurate to call these twins dizygotic (DZ), binovular, or fraternal. But in practice non-identical is a perfectly adequate description.

Since one sperm may carry an X chromosome and another a Y, DZ twins can be of different sexes, and in fact about half of them are. Since two-thirds of all twins are DZ and one half of these are boy-girl pairs, in total a third of all twins are mixed-sex pairs.

DZ twins share half of their genes, on average. Sometimes it's more, sometimes less, which explains why some non-identicals are very similar while others are not at all. They need not have the same father. In 1978, a young German woman gave birth to non-identical boys, one of whom was white and the other black, both conceived on the same day by different men. Actually it's not unusual to find twins of apparently different race. The likeliest cause is not promiscuity, but simply that one or other parent is of mixed racial origin, a situation that provides a rich pool of genes for their children to draw on.

DZ twins are not necessarily conceived on the same day. They can be conceived several days apart, in a phenomenon called superfecundation. This occurs because a woman can be fertile for several days in each menstrual cycle. Perhaps this is why couples with more active sex lives are likelier to have twins. Once in a blue moon, a woman even conceives twins a month or more apart. Normally, a pregnant woman's hormones prevent her from ovulating again until after her baby is born, but in some cases the ovaries go on functioning and release another egg. Debbie Gilbert was the first British woman – and only the fifth in the world – to whom this happened. Tests confirmed that she was already pregnant with daughter Lucy when she conceived son Timothy. Born together in late 1997, at which point Timmy was four weeks premature, the babies were dubbed 'time-lag twins'.

DZ twins can also implant into the womb at different times, sometimes two or more years apart in the case of assisted-fertility techniques where one embryo is frozen for later use. These are twins only in the sense that they were conceived together, and, of course, they will always be of different ages. At Bourn Hall Fertility Clinic, Cambridge, two embryos from the same woman were implanted two years apart into different surrogate mothers, making medical history and resulting in what the tabloid papers called 'time-warp twins'. However, few parents would probably think of them as twins because raising them is no different from bringing up two singletons.

· *What Causes Twins?* ·

I know where a baby comes from, but how did my sister and I get here, Mummy?

Despite a great deal of research into the subject, especially over the last thirty years, the full answer to this question is still largely unknown. There are, however, some important factors which make non-identical, that is DZ, twins more likely. The main factors are:

- race
- family history
- the woman's age
- how many children she already has
- her size and level of nutrition
- increased natural fertility

- fertility treatment
- the contraceptive pill.

The incidence of MZ or identical twins is fairly constant all over the world at about 3.5 per 1,000 maternities (in other words per 1,000 completed pregnancies), but the rate of DZ twinning varies.

Some parts of Africa enjoy the highest rate of twinning on the planet. Compared with her British counterpart, a Nigerian woman of the Yoruba tribe is about four times more likely to have twins. On the other hand, Southeast Asia in general, and Japan in particular, has very low births of DZ twins, although this is now rising because of social changes, including the provision of fertility treatment. White Caucasian women, and Indian Asians, have a DZ twinning rate roughly midway between those two extremes.

Within the UK, area is important too. A few years ago, counties in the affluent south-east of England, such as Surrey, had most twins. This was probably linked to the availability of fertility treatment, and to the fact that mothers there generally delay child-bearing, so that they are older when they become parents. At the moment, Northern Ireland is seeing a huge increase in the number of twins and more. The multiple birth rate in the province has grown by over 50 per cent in 15 years, and now stands at 15.4 in every 1,000 maternities. In 2002, there were 312 sets of twins born, 12 sets of triplets and one set of quins. The reasons are obscure, though the high use of the B vitamin folate in Northern Ireland may have something to do with it. There's no real evidence that folate specifically increases the twinning rate, but quite possibly lowering the incidence of spina bifida may mean that more multiple pregnancies are surviving. Other contenders are minerals in the soil and oestrogens in the water, both strong possibilities since much of Ireland is mountainous.

Twins can run in families. In Australia, the Bauer family had no fewer than 89 sets of twins in five generations. Some women have more than one set of twins. In South Africa, Mrs Barbara Zulu had six sets within seven years. But even she did not break the record set in the nineteenth century by Mrs Mary Jonas, who gave birth to 15 sets of boy-girl twins before dying in 1899, most likely from a combination of shock and exhaustion. Twins are sometimes said to skip a generation, from grandmother to granddaughter, but this isn't true. In reality, a family history of twins makes you more likely to have twins yourself, but it's not inevitable. Some couples with this sort of pedigree like to insure against the possibility of twins. Although twins insurance is now much less common than it once was, it is still possible to shop around and find a broker offering such cover, which could pay out a thousand pounds or more if the woman has twins. There are usually several restrictions, however. The two most usual stipulations are that you take out the policy before the eleventh week of pregnancy, and that you pay the premium before having your first ultrasound scan.

Both the main types of twin may run in families, though it's not certain how. A twinning gene has been found in sheep, but no such luck yet for humans. Research from Sweden shows that any mother who is a twin herself – either MZ or DZ – runs a higher risk of having twins. The genetic factors seem to be completely independent, however: women with DZ twins in the family give birth to more twins of the DZ sort, while those with MZ twins in the family have more MZ twins.

When it comes to making twins, you may think, as many medics do, that only the mother's side of the family matters. After all, men don't ovulate. And in each orgasm a man produces between 150 million and a billion sperms, far more than he needs to produce two babies. Actually, though, research suggests that the male might have a part in conceiving twins after all. It's not certain exactly what happens, but it's possible that sperm can affect the partner's ovum and make it more likely to split into two or more. So there may even be some truth in a father of twins' proud boasts about his virility. This would certainly explain the occasional family in which twins appear to be passed on through the male line. It might not, however, be quite enough to account for the classic Russian story concerning a peasant called Vassilief, who was said to have had two wives in succession and fathered a total of 84 children, amongst them four sets of quads and a staggering seven sets of triplets.

A woman who bears twins is often older. Most twins are born to women aged 25–34, but the likelihood of twins in any one pregnancy is higher in women aged 35–40, because this is when a woman is most likely to produce two eggs at a time. Twin births in this age bracket have rocketed as more and more babies are being born to women in their forties. In a great many developed countries, it's commonplace for women to put off starting a family until they're in their late thirties or even older. As the birth rate among twenty-somethings drops, now more women than ever in their forties are having babies.

The more mature mother may long for a baby, and she often makes an excellent parent, but she's not always so thrilled about the prospect of more than one at a time. Her own relatives may be elderly, so she is less likely to have the benefit of an extended family. Advances in medicine and improvements in social circumstances mean that pregnancy and birth are now safer for the woman over 35, or even 40, than they ever were, but all the same there is still the possibility of health problems, whether related to the pregnancy or not. The mature mother may also find herself sandwiched in a generation of women who have to care for ageing relatives while simultaneously bringing up their own children. On the other hand, the older mother can be mature, socially stable, highly educated and well placed financially to bring up two babies.

A woman pregnant with twins may have several children already; she is what doctors call multiparous. Parity is the number of babies you've had and it increases the likelihood of twins. The more often you play the fruit-machines, the more likely you are to hit the jackpot. She is often taller than average too, and may be heavier. This probably reflects good nutrition rather than anything else – healthy women are more likely to carry two or more babies to a viable age. In the animal kingdom, the reverse applies. Smaller mammals tend to produce most multiples, probably because they are preyed on and therefore need larger litters for the species to survive. Poor nourishment lowers the human twinning rate, so twin births slump during famines and other difficult times.

Natural fertility

Whatever her age, size or state of nutrition, a mother of twins is on average more fertile. According to figures from Canada, Scotland, Denmark and elsewhere, there was a peak in twin births nine months after the end of World War II. This peak actually came two or three months earlier than the post-war baby boom as a whole, suggesting that these women may have found it especially easy to conceive.

Unfortunately, not all women expecting twins intended to have a baby, let alone enjoy the patter of two pairs of tiny feet. In one of her projects, midwifery researcher Jane Spillman found that on average some 16 per cent of mothers of twins had not planned on becoming pregnant yet. Many of these were using contraception, but they fell pregnant all the same.

If you are the mother of twins, you can claim with some pride to be extra fertile. Studies suggest that mothers of twins began their periods at a younger age, have fewer period problems than most women, and their pituitary glands secrete higher levels of follicle-stimulating hormone (FSH). This hormone exerts powerful effects on the ovary, hence some women can produce two eggs in any one cycle. Since FSH levels rise with increasing years, it could explain why age is a risk factor in twinning. Sometimes women who are breast-feeding conceive, despite the natural contraceptive effect of breast-feeding. These women too are more likely to have twins than the average.

The number of daylight hours may play a part by increasing levels of FSH. Regions such as northern Finland and Japan, where the summer brings almost endless light, have reported higher numbers of twin conceptions in July. However, the findings are not conclusive enough to make experts certain on this point.

Staying on the subject of hormones, one theory about the high twinning rate in the Yoruba tribe concerns yams, which are an important part of the diet in rural Nigeria and may exert a hormone-like effect, again increasing FSH levels. Yoruba women who migrate to the big city and adopt a more urban diet tend to leave behind their amazingly high rate of twinning. But it is far from certain that food is the cause.

Worldwide, a possible rebound effect from the contraceptive pill could be significant. It seems that women are more likely to conceive twins in the first month or so after stopping the Pill.

Incidentally, the hormone status of women who have twins may have other interesting consequences. Studies suggest that women who have twins might run a lower risk of breast cancer.

· *What Will Your Twins Be Like?* ·

Will your twins be identical or not? There is an approximate chance of two in three that they will be non-identical (DZ). If your twins are different sexes this clinches it: by definition boy-girl pairs cannot be identical. If they are the same sex, there are a number of helpful clues to look for, though others are misleading.

Many people, including some obstetricians and midwives, still believe that the presence of two placentas means that the twins are non-identical, while one placenta means they are identical. This is not always true. During the pregnancy, two separate placentas can merge and fuse together, while two placentas which are close together may appear to be just one. The membranes attached to the placenta can give more clues. The inner membrane next to a baby is called the amnion, and the outer layer the chorion, as the diagram below shows.

In non-identicals (dizygotic or DZ), about half the twin pairs have a fused placenta, while the rest have two separate placentas. In the one-third of identicals (MZ) who have

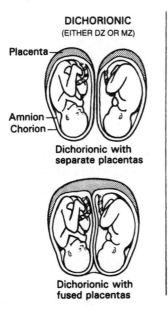
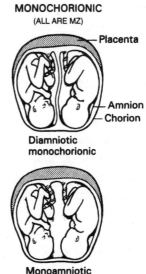

Types of twins and their placentas

dichorionic placentas, these are more likely to be fused, but they too can have separate placentas. Only in identical twins can there be just one chorionic membrane. So if the membranes are carefully examined after delivery and there's only one chorion, the twins must be identical.

What happens in an MZ-twin pregnancy depends on when the fertilised ovum, or zygote, divides into two (there's more on this in the Appendix, page 347).

- If division happens within three days of fertilisation, the twins are dichorionic.
- If it is between three and nine days after fertilisation, they will be monochorionic but diamniotic. In other words, there will still be two separate sacs in the womb.
- If division takes place between nine and 12 days after fertilisation, the twins will be monochorionic and monoamniotic (sharing the same sac). The situation of a forked umbilical cord is very rare, but I have known it happen.
- If it is after 12 days (some experts say 15), the twins could be conjoined.

Siamese (conjoined) twins

Some women worry about the possibility of producing Siamese twins, so called because the original pair of con-joined twins, Chang and Eng, born in 1811, came from Siam (now known as Thailand).

Births of Siamese twins are reported in the media fairly often. Despite several high-profile examples, you can rest assured that they are really very rare. On average, there is perhaps one such pair of twins in every 50,000 to 100,000 pregnancies. Siamese twins are usually picked up by ultrasound scan during pregnancy, or else when the babies are lying in a strange position in the mother's belly.

For some reason, they are more often female than male. The connection between them may be small and insignificant, for instance just a band of tissue at chest level, but occasionally the connection may be more difficult or even impossible to sever without losing one of the twins. Advances in surgery now mean that many more conjoined twins can be successfully separated. However, in rare cases they may share one or more vital organs, such as a heart. Sometimes the connections between them are extensive but still compatible with life, in which case the twins are often able to lead fairly fulfilled lives, including marriage and children. Understandably, compromise between the twins is essential.

· *How Identical are 'Identicals'?* ·

So-called identical or monozygotic (MZ) twins are often described as being like two peas in a pod, but they are rarely indistinguishable. If you look closely, there are always some differences, for instance in their freckles or the shape of the head. And they have different fingerprints, too, although the patterns may be similar. Parents often know the difference even when everyone else is thoroughly baffled.

> *Although my girls are officially identical I've always been able to tell them apart, except in photos taken as tiny babies when I can't remember who wore what! Rachel and Zoe just look and sound different to me and even feel different. If one of them pads into the bedroom in the night for a hug, I can always tell who it is!*

However understandable it may be, it is a mistake to think of MZ twins as exactly alike. Your 'identical' youngsters could, for instance, have different personalities. Even from an early age their hair may curl in opposite directions at the nape of the neck, they may lie in completely different positions in their cots, their cries may be dissimilar, and they may very soon like different foods. They share the same genetic material, but environment has a great deal to answer for too. At first glance one might expect twins to share the same environment, but they do not necessarily, or rather not in every detail.

Subtle differences at crucial times could make a huge impact later. The fetal origins hypothesis is now widely accepted, at least for singletons. According to this theory, circumstances before birth can programme a human for the rest of his life, altering his physiology for ever.

Nobody is quite sure how early programming might apply to twins, but experts have come up with suggestions. For a start, MZ twins can get different amounts of blood from the placenta, which is why they often have dissimilar birth weights. Even babies sharing a forked umbilical cord get different amounts of blood through it. Position in the womb might be important; for instance, the mother's heartbeat might be much louder for one twin during a critical period of maturation. Infections during pregnancy can affect one twin and not the other. All these early differences could prove vitally important later. And of course one twin is always born before the other, even during a caesarean birth, so the experience during delivery could be crucially dissimilar even for identical twins.

The genes may be the same for each twin, but genes are not always switched on. Even identical twins do not necessarily both get, say, asthma, hay fever or food allergies, conditions which are widely viewed as genetic. There are mechanisms that effectively silence several genes. In fact a whole chromosome can be switched off. Chromosome inactivation refers to the fact that one chromosome can lie dormant. This is known to happen to one X chromosome in girls, and it explains why even some conditions like muscular dystrophy, which are definitely genetic and inherited on the X chromosome, do not necessarily affect both 'identical' twins.

I said identical twins share the same genes, but this may not be entirely true. There is now even evidence that MZ twins need not be genetically identical, because there could be errors in chromosome splitting. Or, after the split, minor changes to DNA (deoxyribonucleic acid) could occur. DNA may be the building blocks of life, but even the hardest bricks can get the odd chip.

With some MZ twin pairs, one twin is right-handed while the other is left-handed. Some researchers claim that up to a third of MZ twins are left-handed, which is about double the rate in the general population. It's not certain what makes a human favour one hand over the other, so it is no surprise that the origins of handedness in twins are hotly debated. Some think that birth stress or low birth weight is relevant to handedness – or laterality, as medics sometimes call it. But the cause, whatever it is, probably goes back much further than that: on ultrasound scans as early as nine or ten weeks of pregnancy, a tiny fetus shows a preference for one arm or the other.

Mirror-imaging is something you may hear about. Harmless but fascinating, this could affect up to a quarter of identical twins. In mirror-image twins, hair patterns, handedness and fingerprints can be reversed, literally as if seen in a mirror. This is not necessarily linked with any internal disorders, such as situs inversus, in which major organs are shifted from left to right and vice versa. In fact, it usually causes no problems at all, other than those of a purely practical nature. If, for instance, you seat a left-handed child on the right of a right-handed child at a table, do not be surprised if neither of them can write, draw or eat very easily. The cause of mirror-imaging is, as you might have guessed, yet another mystery at the moment. It could be due to late splitting of the fertilised ovum, after right and left sides are already established.

Zygosity – identical or not?

If you have a same-sex pair, they may be very alike, just like two sisters or brothers can be. You can get a good idea of your twins' identicalness (or zygosity, as it's scientifically known) by looking closely at some of your babies' features. Identical twins can differ in weight, height and shape of head, but they have the same:

- hair colour
- eye colour
- skin colour.

They also have the same blood group. So, if your twins are dissimilar in any of these respects, they are not identical (there are only a very few exceptions). The shape of the ears is said to be quite a useful indicator, as it is less likely to be affected by position in the womb than is the head shape as a whole; ears, therefore, tend to look the same in MZ twins. In fact, ear shapes are so significant that research is in progress on the possibility of mapping digital ear scans with a view to linking them to DNA fingerprinting.

Fairly simple laboratory tests – looking at the placenta and membranes and checking blood groups – are up to 80 per cent accurate in determining identicalness (zygosity). If you have same-sex twins and they have only one chorionic membrane (see page 23) then they must be identical. But if they don't, how will you know for sure?

DNA fingerprinting

DNA (deoxyribonucleic acid) is the complex protein that

carries the genetic code and is sometimes referred to as the blueprint or the building block of life. DNA fingerprinting is a way of testing for many different DNA characteristics at the same time and is the most accurate way of finding out if your twins are identical (MZ). The laboratory can examine specific regions of your children's genetic codes and compare the patterns against each other. MZ twins have the same DNA fingerprints, while non-identical (DZ) twins have one chance in about 3×10^{14} of being the same; that's a probability of one in 300,000,000,000,000, so you can consider the test to be pretty conclusive. However, it can give completely misleading results if done within a few months of a blood transfusion.

DNA fingerprinting is a technique used in forensic science and it can be done on an individual's hair, skin, saliva or semen. It can also be carried out on the placenta or a small amount of a baby's cord blood, and even on a stillborn baby if need be. Strange as it may sound, DNA testing is actually more accurate when it is done on skin or saliva than on blood. In practice, a swab from inside the cheek is the usual method for checking the zygosity of twins.

Getting it done is not that simple, alas. DNA testing is expensive and you may have to pay for it yourself unless you're in the tiny minority who have a strong medical case for needing to know (for example, if one of your twins needs a transplant). Should you want to get it done, you can contact the Multiple Births Foundation (MBF) for details of a testing service. You may need to use a private laboratory via the internet, and send cheek swabs through the post. At the time of writing you can expect to pay in the region of £80–90 for testing your twins. No medical test, not even a zygosity test, can give an answer that you can rely on 100 per cent. This test is around 99.99 per cent accurate, which is more than good enough for most of us.

Does it really matter if your twins are identical? Well, it

may be important if you are contemplating another pregnancy, since you are slightly more likely to have a second set
of twins if the first set was DZ. Parents often like to know
anyway, even if their family is complete. A study done for the
MBF confirms that most mothers do consider it important,
yet of the mothers interviewed, over half had been given
inaccurate information, based on incorrect assumptions
about the placenta and zygosity (see page 348 on placentas
and chorionicity). If they had merely taken random guesses,
they'd have been right half the time. In fact, these mothers
would have done better had they simply tossed a coin!

*I don't know if my boys are identical or not. I don't really mind
one way or the other. But people do ask and I feel stupid not being
able to give an accurate answer. Besides, my sons have started to
ask if they came from the same egg.*

· *Twins and Growth* ·

Interestingly, there tends to be a greater discrepancy in birth
weight between identical twins than non-identical twins,
because in the womb identicals often share a blood supply
unequally, as I've already mentioned.

Even when there are marked differences in weight or
height, in the case of identicals these usually even up as the
years pass. A few identical twins don't equalise, and they're
often the ones who were affected by twin-to-twin transfusion
syndrome (TTTS, see Appendix, page 348). Non-identicals
tend to differ more as they grow up and there is no more
reason for them to be the same size than there is for any
other two siblings. It is just that when children are exactly
the same age the differences are more obvious. Same-sex
pairs are usually more alike as adults than are boy-girl pairs.

Twins generally grow just as tall as singletons, though

studies show that they are often a bit thinner. They tend to grow especially quickly as babies. By the age of nine, twins have almost caught up in height with singletons. Both MZ and DZ twins are of average height but tend to be below the average weight for the population (probably no bad thing). Paediatrician Dr John Buckler, an expert in the growth of multiples, points out that this may mean that in adulthood the twins will be somewhat shorter than their parents; as mentioned earlier, parents of twins tend to be taller than average. For the same reason, twins are often smaller in stature than their non-twin siblings too.

Girl twins, for some mysterious reason, often achieve comparatively greater height than boys, but even so the boy will, as a man, be on average 13 cm (5 inches) taller than his twin sister. The growth of triplets is believed to be similar to that of twins, but much less information is available here.

· *Intelligence* ·

It is sometimes said that twins are less bright than singletons, and many studies do show that IQ (intelligence quotient), as measured in formal tests, tends to be a few points lower in twins. However, a few points rarely matter in everyday life – or even in academic life. These average findings tell you nothing about your own twins, either (or both) of whom may be on a par with geniuses. There is no evidence of any significant difference between twins and singletons in general intelligence. Nor should you assume, if you have other children, that they will be brighter than your twins, or more likely to succeed in life. Common sense and what's sometimes called emotional intelligence are far more important ingredients.

Twins can differ from each other intellectually and developmentally. One of the longest-running studies is the ongoing Louisville Twin Study in Kentucky. It began over 30 years ago and looks at both the physical and mental development of twins, assessing these not just as snapshots at any one point in time, but looking at how the measurements change over a matter of years. Work from Louisville and elsewhere suggests that, as with height and weight, MZ twins tend to perform in a similar way in IQ tests, and continue to do so as time passes, while DZ pairs become less alike as the years go by. Even so, it would be unfair of a parent to assume from this research that their MZ twins have to have similar IQ scores.

One interesting finding is that the IQ of boy-girl pairs is more similar than that of same-sex DZ pairs. But why? Perhaps because same-sex pairs need to go to great lengths to express their individuality, while boy-girl pairs don't have to: the differences between them are obvious enough not to need emphasising by behaving in dissimilar ways.

This brings me to the interplay between genetics and the environment, something which is at the centre of the debate about nature versus nurture in general and the study of twins in particular. Take reading, for instance. Researchers at the Institute of Child Health, London, studying language problems in twins – a topic explored in Chapter 10 – have confirmed that identicals tend to have similar language delays, whereas non-identicals do not. Part of the explanation may lie in the fact that identicals share the same genes. But they often share more than that, since they are more likely to be treated as one unit than non-identical twins are. For example, a parent is more apt to read to young children together, or to address them simultaneously, if they look very alike. So it is not always easy to tease out the relative contributions of genes and the environment.

A huge amount of work is going on in these and other areas pertaining to multiples. One organisation responsible for bringing together all kinds of scientists in the field of twin work is the International Society for Twin Studies, formed in 1974 by the geneticist Professor Luigi Gedda, and based, appropriately enough, in Rome, the city said to have been founded by Romulus. The society's official journal, *Twin Research*, was launched in 1998 and is published six times a year. Although most of the publication has little to offer non-scientists, there are occasionally articles that could interest parents of twins.

· *Triplets and More* ·

What if you are having triplets or even higher multiples? First of all, if you are expecting three or more babies, you are slightly more likely to have more girls than boys. The more babies you produce at once, the higher will be the proportion of girls. About 51 per cent of all single-born babies – but only 46 per cent of quadruplets – are male.

Like twins, triplets can arise in more than one way. They are often trizygotic – developing from three fertilised ova. Sometimes they are dizygotic (from two ova, one of which splits to form a monozygotic pair, which are therefore identical). On rare occasions, they can be monozygotic (one fertilised egg splits and one of those halves splits again).

Much the same applies – though in a more complicated way – to higher-order births. The Dionne quintuplets, born in Canada in the 1930s, are believed to be identical (MZ).

Whenever I was out with my three (two girls and a boy), I'd be asked how they were conceived. I thought they were ignorant, and wondered if I was supposed to draw them a picture. But then of course I realised that they wanted to know if they were test tube babies or all our own work.

· Infertility Treatment and · Multiple Births

Less than a third of triplet and higher-order births are conceived in the old-fashioned biblical way, the rest being due to various forms of infertility treatment. Almost all quads and above are the outcome of assisted-fertility techniques. This is an estimate, as no country officially records the way multiples are conceived, but it goes some way to explaining the phenomenal rise in triplets in the last couple of decades.

In vitro fertilisation (IVF) – only one of several techniques – has led to the birth of over 68,000 children in the UK since the first 'test-tube baby', Louise Brown, in 1978. IVF now accounts for 1 per cent of all births in Britain.

Assisted-conception techniques raise all sorts of complex ethical questions, many of which – like sex selection and the fate of frozen embryos – are outside the scope of this book. Looking simply at the practical aspects, it is obvious that large numbers of multiple births, together with the medical advances which enable more tiny babies to survive, put huge pressure on hospital services.

As one obstetrician in training put it:

A few years back, I was going around the Special Care Baby Unit early one morning, when I realised that it was literally full of triplets. In terms of our methods in the infertility clinic, I began to think of multiple pregnancy less as a success and more as a disaster.

Fertility problems are said to affect one couple in every six, increasing numbers of whom seek help for their difficulties in conceiving. Worldwide, various assisted-reproduction techniques are responsible for a 20 to 33 per cent risk of twins or higher-order births. In 2001, about 27 per cent of IVF pregnancies in the UK led to twins or more.

At first sight, IVF does seem to be the likeliest culprit for the rise in multiple births with infertility treatments. In this technique, the woman is given drugs to make her release as many eggs as possible. Her eggs are then collected, fertilised in the laboratory and finally replaced (transferred) as embryos directly into her womb.

To maximise the chances of success, the received wisdom has been to implant more than one embryo into the womb, but how many is the right number? Too few and the technique could fail. Too many and many multiple pregnancies could result. This is how most quads and high multiples arise, and there is an increased risk of losing one or more of the embryos, perhaps even all of them.

Infertility clinics are becoming more skilled, and at the same time increasingly aware, that replacing fewer embryos can actually give a better success rate, if you consider the end-point that really matters to prospective parents – not the raw figures for numbers of pregnancies achieved by the clinic, but the take-home-baby rate.

Incidentally, IVF produces multiples from different ova, at least in theory. In practice, it sometimes results in multiples which are identical (MZ) too, which means that triplets from IVF are not always trizygotic. Fertility specialists now believe that something changes in the outer layer (called the zona pellucida) of the ovum during the process of IVF, so that the covering becomes more brittle and thus more likely to divide to produce two identical embryos. An early embryo can actually split into two when prodded by a glass rod in the laboratory during the process of embryo transfer.

In Britain, IVF is regulated by the Human Fertilisation and Embryology Authority (HFEA), a non-departmental government body set up in 1991. The HFEA maintains a clinic register, and regulates and inspects all clinics which use IVF or donor sperm or eggs, or which store eggs, sperm or embryos. This may sound all-encompassing, but it is not.

Until recently, no more than three embryos could be replaced in each IVF procedure, and since 2001 that limit has gone down to two. The change in policy was meant to encourage good practice in fertility clinics and to reduce the soaring number of multiple births. With the launch of the HFEA's sixth code of practice in 2004, only women over 40 may have three embryos transferred in a single cycle. In fact, transferring two embryos can reduce the triplet rate from 6 per cent to 0.4 per cent, very welcome news to all those expectant parents who have only two arms apiece. The time will probably come when results from IVF are more reliable and single-embryo transfer becomes the norm. This is already the case in Denmark and Sweden, for example, while in the USA the transfer of large numbers of embryos is still routine.

HFEA figures for 2001 reveal that women treated in over 100 infertility clinics gave birth to 4,621 single babies, 3,158 twins and 327 triplets. IVF may now be the best-regulated fertility technique in Britain, but it is not the only method. There is also donor insemination, which is also regulated by the HFEA. Then there is GIFT (gamete intra-fallopian transfer), IUI (intra-uterine insemination) and ovulation induction. Any medics with the know-how could perform these without a special licence from the HFEA because they do not involve fertilisation of eggs outside the body, or donation or storage of eggs or sperm. These methods too can produce multiple births. It's estimated that GIFT involves a multiple pregnancy rate of around 7 per cent. At the moment, the sobering reality is that the HFEA is not even sure how many of these procedures are done every year.

Drugs which bring on ovulation are a relatively low-tech treatment for infertility and are easy to administer, but they can cause problems if given without proper monitoring. A woman may not know, until it's too late, that she has produced two, three, or even more eggs in one cycle instead of the required one.

I resented it deeply. Yes, I got pregnant when I wanted, but all I asked for was one baby at a time.

Some well-meaning GPs and hospital doctors prescribe ovulation-inducing drugs in this way. It is a much quicker method of achieving a pregnancy than waiting for an appointment at a specialist clinic, and the doctors' motives may be laudable, but it is now clear that inducing ovulation with drugs can do women a disservice unless the treatment is carefully monitored to check how many eggs are produced.

Couples undergoing treatment for fertility problems need to know the risk of multiple pregnancy. The HFEA even makes it obligatory for every centre performing IVF to offer counselling, so that would-be parents appreciate that they could have twins, triplets, or more. However, there can be a wide gulf between hearing what is said and absorbing all the practical implications.

A couple may be so desperate for a child that multiple pregnancy seems a small price to pay and they are likely to underestimate the risk as well as the potential problems. Older women especially may feel that time is running out. Others may even welcome the thought of an instant family, particularly if they are making huge sacrifices to fund their treatment, as many do when unable to obtain it on the NHS.

Quite apart from the cost of the treatment itself, bringing up babies is expensive. In 2003, the insurance group AXA estimated that the total cost of raising one child from birth to the age of 21 came to £300,000. You can deduct £139,000 if you send your child to state schools, but you still need around £22,000 for clothing, £35,000 for food and £27,000 for university education. Getting down to specifics, *Prima Baby* magazine has calculated that a woman loses around £9,000 of earnings while she is on maternity leave. If she returns to work, she can expect more expense, and the cost of childcare often increases with each additional child.

You also need to duplicate almost everything (except for obvious items like baby baths) for each baby born at the same time, making multiples an expensive proposition. Some families need a bigger car or a larger home. Many are forced to consider building an extension or taking on a larger mortgage at a time when finances are particularly tight. Statutory help is not always enough. Tax credits were introduced in 2003 for parents. The child tax credit helps most parents, while the working tax credit helps those with lower incomes. Parents with a child under 12 months of age can get an additional payment, but the snag for those reading this book is that parents of multiples get this only once, which is unfair. Tamba is campaigning to get rid of this inequality.

Setting aside the potential impact on a family's emotional and financial resources if one or more babies has special needs and requires extra provision, even healthy multiples exact a high manpower cost. It has been estimated by a mother of triplets that babycare and related household chores eat up 197½ hours per week, a schedule that would stagger even a junior hospital doctor. Since there are only 168 hours in a week, extra help has to be enlisted (and funded), or many tasks must be dropped altogether.

It is not easy going through assisted-fertility treatment, and when it produces multiples a couple can have a hard time acknowledging the difficulties they face. This is the hoped-for parenthood – to whom can they admit their doubts? Can they own up to not being perfect? People are not always sympathetic and may even tell a couple that they have brought their troubles on themselves. The challenges aren't insuperable, but it can be hard. Tamba runs an Infertility Support Group which can help parents deal with these and other issues, as well as Supertwins and Special Needs groups.

Chapter Two
YOUR MULTIPLE PREGNANCY

I just knew something was different and soon after my pregnancy test was positive I wondered if it was twins. I was feeling a lot sicker than with my first baby, though a doctor friend of mine said I was probably just having a girl this time. The junior doctor in the clinic didn't believe me either. She sent me for a scan, having written on the form 'to exclude twins'. I left the clinic thinking, 'What rubbish – surely she means "to confirm twins".'

Being pregnant with two or more babies often feels different from being pregnant with one. Until about 26 weeks into the pregnancy, the growth of each twin (and possibly each triplet) is roughly the same as that of a single baby. This means that at any one stage of pregnancy your bump is more impressive. In a twin pregnancy, your womb is the same volume and size as that of a woman expecting a single baby who is up to eight weeks nearer her due date. For instance at 20 weeks, the fundus (the top end) of the womb can be felt at 20 cm (8 inches) above the pubic bone in a singleton pregnancy, but if you're expecting twins, your fundus is likely to be higher by 4 cm (1½ inches) or more. By the time you get to 28 weeks, you could be looking and feeling nearly as large as a woman carrying one baby at term.

By the time you get to term, the volume of your womb could be nearly twice as big. Studies show that at term the inner volume of the uterus is 5 litres (about 9 pints) with singletons and nearly 10 litres (17½ pints) with twins! And with triplets, you're likely to be 10 or 12 weeks greater in size as compared with a mum of singletons.

> *When I was expecting Ben and Sam, I was gigantic. Something poked under my ribs constantly from about 30 weeks and the side view in the mirror was alarming – I've kept photos to prove it. By 37 weeks I could hardly sit with my legs together because the bump took so much room.*

Fortunately, you probably won't be pregnant for quite as long as with a singleton.

- While 40 weeks is 'full term' for a single baby, 37 weeks is considered to be full term for twins.
- For triplets, the average length of gestation is 34 weeks.
- For quads, it is 32 weeks – nearly two months shorter than a singleton pregnancy.

Premature labour, when the babies arrive earlier than anticipated, is one of the main hazards of twin and higher-order pregnancies. This is covered in Chapter 3, and it is well worth reading this soon, so that you know what signs to look out for and what to do about them. Other symptoms and complications which can be commoner in multiple pregnancy are covered here, along with the important physical and emotional adjustments you need to make before your babies arrive.

Twice as pregnant?

A few women carrying multiples just know, in some cases long before their first scan, that they are carrying more than one baby. You may need to wear your maternity clothes a lot earlier than you expected (although this is common in second and subsequent pregnancies anyway, because the abdominal muscles are weaker by then). Later on, you may notice that you are a slightly different shape, with a definite bulge towards the sides, not just the front. You may also feel more kicks than with one baby.

> *Before the scan confirmed twins, I was grilled by the midwife in the clinic who assumed I was just further on in my pregnancy than I thought. She asked me several times if I was sure of my 'dates', i.e. of my last period, which I was. In fact, as an accountant, I was somewhat insulted by her apparent accusation and I retorted huffily that I knew not only the days of the week but also the months of the year.*

· *Weight Changes* ·

Weight gain in pregnancy varies, not just according to how well your babies are growing, but also on whether you were overweight to start with. Some women put on almost 25 kg (4 stone) while carrying twins, though most gain less than this. How much you should gain – and when – is hard to say, especially with quads and other higher-order births, because there are just not enough of them born to work out a useful guide. However, a number of studies taken together suggest that a good or 'recommended' weight gain would be:

- For a twin pregnancy, a total gain of 18–23 kg (40–50lb), preferably 11 kg (24 lb) by week 24, and then 0.6 kg (1¼ lb) a week until birth.
- For triplets, a total gain of 23–27 kg (50–60 lb), preferably 16 kg (36 lb) by week 24, then 0.6 kg (1¼ lb) a week until birth.
- For quads, a total gain of 31–36 kg (68–80 lb), again ideally with most of the weight increase by week 24.

Why the emphasis on early weight gain? The theory is that

the better nourished you are in early pregnancy, the better your babies will grow during the vital time when organs are formed, and the fitter they'll be at birth. Research from the USA suggests that with twins, early weight gain means a better final outcome, with perhaps fewer babies going into the Special Care Baby Unit, but it's not universally accepted.

Nutrition in the womb is important, though it's not clear in exactly what ways. In Chapter 1, I mentioned the fetal origins hypothesis, and it is fascinating. At the moment, one can't be certain that the theory applies to twins. In the womb, twins are often smaller in size than singletons, but there's conflicting evidence as to whether it's a disadvantage for later health in terms of heart disease and related problems like high blood pressure, high cholesterol and diabetes. A lot of research is going on.

You may be horrified at the thought of gaining a lot of weight in this pregnancy, especially if you already feel you have a weight problem, or you have always struggled to stay slim. You do need to put on weight, though, for the sake of your babies. Later in this chapter, on the section Caring for Yourself During Pregnancy, you'll find concrete guidance on what to eat when you're expecting twins or more, so that you can be sure that what you eat is put to good use inside your growing uterus.

· *Other Bodily Changes* ·

Along with increasing bulk go a number of inner changes. The way a woman's body adapts to carrying more than one fetus at a time has not been nearly as well studied as the average singleton pregnancy, but there are some well-known changes.

Heart and circulation

In the mother's circulation, the volume of blood (or to be exact the volume of plasma, which is the blood minus all the cells carried in it) begins to expand in the first three months of pregnancy. It rises rapidly in the second three months and continues to increase, although more slowly, to reach a plateau a few weeks before birth. So, if you are carrying just one baby, your final maximum blood volume in pregnancy is nearly 50 per cent greater than it was before you were pregnant. In a twin pregnancy, however, the staggering fact is that its maximum is nearly double your pre-pregnant level (not that you will notice it – the increase is all inside the blood vessels).

To cope with the increase in blood volume and pump it around the bloodstream, your heart will have to work a lot harder in a multiple pregnancy. Your blood pressure will drop, which is normal in pregnancy, and your pulse rate will rise to keep the circulation going. This won't matter much unless you already happen to have heart trouble, or plan to take strenuous exercise in late pregnancy. In practical terms, this means you should not play squash, for instance, towards the end of your twin pregnancy, although you probably won't feel like it anyway. There's more on rest and exercise later in this chapter. If you have any queries as to how much sport you can or cannot play, check with your doctor.

Anaemia

Carrying more than one baby uses up a mother's reserves of both iron and folic acid, as well as other vitamins. It is estimated that a pregnant woman needs an extra 570 mg of iron for herself during pregnancy, plus around 430 mg for each fetus. In fact, a woman's stores of iron are often low in a multiple pregnancy, though this is not a test that is done routinely in pregnancy.

A woman who is well nourished herself can often handle the extra demands of twin pregnancy without becoming anaemic. Experts don't all agree on iron. Some obstetricians recommend iron tablets routinely in pregnancy for mums of multiples, others don't. You should be taking folate already, and continue to take it until 13 weeks. If you are given iron tablets and you are not sure if you really need them, ask your doctor or midwife. In some case you may be able to avoid iron, which may spare you the constipation that can result.

Obviously, if you were to develop anaemia, you would need treatment (usually with tablets, but sometimes by injection). Anaemia is one of the conditions which show up on routine antenatal blood tests, and your records will show your Hb (haemoglobin) level. However, Hb should not be taken at face value: it is normal for it to drop, but this is because the blood volume expands, as explained above. After 20 weeks, for instance, the average Hb in a twin pregnancy is around 10 g/dl (the normal Hb level is 12 to 14), not necessarily because the woman is getting dangerously anaemic but because the red blood cells are swimming in a larger volume. It is one of the other figures in the blood result (the average Hb concentration per cell) that shows whether true anaemia is present. If your Hb drops, you will have a further blood test to make sure exactly why this happened.

· *Symptoms of Pregnancy* ·

Many women feel at their best in pregnancy, while others find this supposedly joyous time marred by symptoms such as:

- nausea or vomiting
- heartburn

- constipation
- headache
- varicose veins
- piles
- backache
- sleeplessness.

In practice these can be quite troublesome, yet they are still considered minor problems (and often dismissed by doctors) because they are not medically serious. They are caused mainly by the sheer size of the enlarging uterus, the hormones of pregnancy, or the way your body is adapting. The better a placenta functions, the more hormones it makes. So, in many cases, the worse the symptoms, the stronger the babies are growing. No wonder medics can remain unimpressed by a list of pregnancy-related complaints. There are tips on how to care for yourself and cope with pregnancy symptoms later in this chapter.

· *Medical Complications* ·

Aches and pains apart, multiple pregnancy tends to be more complicated from the purely medical angle. The possibility of complications, however remote it may seem to you, is one very good reason for antenatal care.

A twin or higher-order pregnancy is not the norm for humans, something mothers-to-be (and those caring for them) need to remember. The extra risk involved in a twin pregnancy is a fact you just have to accept, regardless of how easy or straightforward any previous pregnancy may have been. While there is no need to lie awake worrying about what could go wrong, don't get too blasé either.

This should be a happy and enjoyable time for you. You should be able to revel in your increasing size, and look forward to the delights in store once your babies arrive. However, because there is a risk of complications, you need to attend the antenatal clinic a little more often and have more frequent scans. You can still expect to have a named midwife or midwife team, but you may find that you see more health professionals at your clinic visits. This is not just because twins are more interesting to doctors and midwives, but because teamwork is an important ingredient of effective antenatal care and a good way of ensuring the best outcome for you and your babies.

Although it's worth emphasising that most women sail through their multiple pregnancy without any of the following complications, statistically there is a higher risk of:

- vaginal bleeding (including miscarriage, placental abruption and antepartum haemorrhage)
- poor growth of one or more babies
- pre-eclampsia (toxaemia; see page 47)
- hydramnios (see page 49)
- twin-to-twin transfusion syndrome (see Appendix, page 348).
- premature labour (see Chapter 3).

I sincerely apologise if any readers are put off or even alarmed by the explanations below. You can always skip them if you don't want to read them. However, like many other doctors, I firmly believe that being aware of the possibilities is to be forearmed and could even save your babies' lives.

Vaginal bleeding

This is said to be nearly three times more common in twin than single pregnancy, though precise figures are hard to come by and the exact cause is unknown. Some women get minor bleeding when the fertilised eggs implant into the womb, and women who conceive twins or more can get a heavier implantation bleed. This occurs in the first two weeks of pregnancy, around the time of the first missed period. Later in pregnancy, women with twins or more are again more likely to experience bleeding. One might expect a higher incidence of placenta praevia (where one or other placenta lies very low in the womb) purely because in a multiple pregnancy more of the uterus is taken up by placentas, but this doesn't wholly explain the extra risk of bleeding in twin or higher-order pregnancies.

Bleeding in pregnancy actually comes from the wall of the womb, not from the babies. All the same, the heavier the blood loss, the more likely it is to be serious, as you might guess. Many women who bleed in pregnancy will eventually deliver normal babies, but you can't assume this at the time. Always contact your doctor or midwife without delay if you bleed while pregnant, and expect to have a scan to assess the situation.

Pre-eclampsia

I had read about pre-eclampsia but didn't realise it was more common with twins. Although I had swelling from early pregnancy, nobody diagnosed pre-eclampsia until it was so bad I was admitted to hospital at a routine 32-week appointment. I was upset that I wasn't prepared for the babies, but with hindsight I know how important it was to be closely monitored. When my blood pressure went sky high at 34 weeks, my baby girls were delivered by caesarean. Though small, they were absolutely fine.

This potentially lethal condition is more common in twin and multiple pregnancies. Not all pregnant women have even heard of pre-eclampsia (also known as toxaemia of pregnancy, or PET), yet it is the commonest cause of maternal death in Britain and it can also kill one or both babies, so it's worth taking seriously. If you already have high blood pressure or kidney disease, you're more likely to develop it.

PET is more common in a primigravida (first-time mum) and is thought to be due to some abnormality of the placenta, or placentas. It is not clear quite what the problem is and studies are under way in order to understand and treat PET better. Research from Oxford shows that normal pregnancy can trigger an inflammatory reaction which goes into over-drive in women with pre-eclampsia. A larger placenta causes an exaggerated inflammatory response, which may be why multiple pregnancies are more likely to lead to PET. There's currently research into the possibility that certain vitamins could cut the risk, but for the moment there's no way of preventing it.

Pre-eclampsia seems to be a multi-organ disorder, and can cause liver problems and blood-clotting abnormalities in the mother. The kidneys don't function properly either, so the babies aren't nourished as well as normal. Not surprisingly, PET affects the growth of the fetus or fetuses.

The condition can come on any time after 20 weeks of pregnancy, and causes raised blood pressure in the mother and makes her lose protein in the urine. Fluid retention is also a symptom of pre-eclampsia, but this is sometimes hard to spot since puffy hands and feet are common in late preg-nancy. However, puffiness and swelling are more marked in PET.

Picking up PET early is one of the most important reasons for keeping antenatal appointments. Blood pressure, urine and weight should be checked each time (though the last measurement seems to be going out of favour). Along with many other doctors, I believe the possibility of PET is a compelling argument against further cuts in antenatal care. If anything, some pregnant women should be checked more often, in accordance with new British guidelines on diagnosing and treating pre-eclampsia.

PET is about three to five times more common in twin pregnancies. Mild forms of PET affect about a fifth of all first-time mothers expecting singletons and about a quarter of those expecting twins. Smoking seems to increase the risk of PET. Severe PET is less common than the uncomplicated form of the condition, but it can develop into eclampsia. Typically, a woman with eclampsia has fits (convulsions) and sometimes lasting kidney damage. In multiple pregnancies, PET is often more severe and comes on earlier – or progresses more rapidly. That's why it makes sense to know something about it, and for doctors and midwives to act on any suspicions they may have.

If PET is diagnosed, the priority is usually to deliver the baby or babies, assuming they are mature enough to survive happily outside the womb. Deciding when to deliver is a little more difficult with multiples than it is with singletons, but the general principles of treatment are exactly the same. Sometimes treating raised blood pressure in its own right can help treat PET. In severe PET and eclampsia, magnesium sulphate injections can relieve or prevent fits.

Hydramnios

Hydramnios (also called polyhydramnios) is excess amniotic fluid, often to the point where it becomes uncomfortable for the woman, as well as being more difficult for the doctor or midwife to feel the fetus.

Hydramnios affects around 5 per cent of multiple pregnancies and tends to develop in the last third of pregnancy. Draining off some of the fluid can make the mother more comfortable. On the other hand, there is some risk that this will trigger premature labour without treating the underlying cause of the excess fluid in the first place. Sometimes taking drugs like the anti-inflammatory drug indomethacin helps, but this needs to be under medical supervision, as it can have side-effects for the babies.

The real importance of hydramnios is that it can be linked with other complications, in particular twin-to-twin transfusion syndrome (see Appendix, page 348), gestational diabetes (diabetes in pregnancy), and severe forms of pre-eclampsia. Therefore, if you seem to have too much amniotic fluid, you will probably be sent for another ultrasound scan to check everything is all right.

· *Ultrasound Scans* ·

Ultrasound scans (USS) use waves of the same type as sound. When they first came in, it was assumed that they were completely safe because they use no X-rays, but in the last few years some people have had doubts about both the increasing role of USS and its safety. Really conclusive answers are not available, which isn't surprising, as one can't often prove absence of risk. However, you can be sure that no significant problems have emerged since the early 1970s, when antenatal ultrasound first became widely used.

One objection to routine use of technology like USS is that it can over-medicalise a pregnancy, but ultrasound scanning has undoubtedly been a boon to pregnant women and those who care for them. Among other things, USS can:

- ensure a baby is growing in the uterus, not one of the fallopian tubes
- confirm the expected date of delivery
- help in managing bleeding during pregnancy
- locate the placenta (for instance, diagnosing placenta praevia)

- estimate the amount of amniotic fluid
- pick up congenital abnormalities
- enable tests like amniocentesis and chorionic villus sampling (CVS), and interventions like fetal blood transfusion, to be done safely
- identify breech babies before labour (this can affect the method of delivery).

Using a form of scan called Doppler ultrasound, it is also possible to assess blood flow in the umbilical arteries and in the baby's heart, so it can be a good measure of an unborn baby's wellbeing.

In multiple pregnancies, USS is even more useful, as it can:

- detect twin and higher-order pregnancies in the first place
- monitor the growth of each baby
- pick up abnormalities in cases where blood tests cannot help
- detect which twin pregnancies are at especially high risk (see the section on chorionicity in the Appendix)
- diagnose complications of pregnancy, such as polyhydramnios (see page 49) and twin-to-twin transfusion syndrome (see Appendix, page 348)
- visualise the state of the cervix to assess the risk of premature birth
- observe the interaction of twins before birth (see Chapter 9).

Diagnosing multiples

Your first contact with the USS department may well be momentous, since this is probably when you will discover (officially) that you are expecting more than one baby. Actually, all first scans carried out in pregnancy should check for twins because not every woman has symptoms or a family tree suggesting that she is likely to have multiples. Usually the first scan is at around 13–14 weeks, but may be much earlier if, for instance:

- you have fertility treatment
- you are unsure of the date of your last period
- you have symptoms such as bleeding.

Many departments can pick up twins and more with nearly 100 per cent accuracy, so the days when over half of all twins came as a surprise in the delivery suite are, thankfully, long gone. But twins can still be missed if a scan is done very early (much before 12 weeks), especially with an inexperienced sonographer, as the USS technician is called.

Occasionally triplets have been misdiagnosed. About 6 per cent of triplets and 16 per cent of quads are not spotted until scans later in pregnancy. It is unusual, though not unknown, for the news 'It's twins' to be upgraded to 'It's triplets' on the next scan and even to quads on a subsequent scan . . .

For most women, the exciting fact that they're having twins comes as an exhilarating surprise, while for others it is a huge shock to the system. Unfortunately, the way in which they get the news can sometimes create distress.

The technician just frowned at the screen and muttered darkly under her breath. She didn't seem to hear me when I asked if everything was OK. She only said that she'd have to get a colleague in and wouldn't be long. I lay there and my life flashed before me. I just knew it: my baby was deformed. The news just cut everything in two: before and after. I was in shock. The technician came back with someone else after what seemed like ages and then I was told I was having twins. It was such a relief, but I could hardly believe it.

It may seem unreal to begin with, and while you are on your way home you may begin to doubt whether you heard right.

Many USS departments can, for a small fee, give you a photo of the scan to keep. At home, you can pore over this with your partner, which can help you get used to the idea of two (or more) babies. However, whether you have a picture or not, your first scan is likely to be the moment that begins your lifelong relationship with your children.

It would be nice if staff could help answer queries about twins soon after the scan, but often this is not possible. However, just after you leave the USS department is a good time to get in touch with Tamba, if you haven't already; many women are hugely reassured by being given the number for their local twins' club or for Tamba Twinline by the hospital staff directly after their scan confirms twins.

Monitoring growth

Other things being equal, the larger the bump, the better the baby is growing, but in a twin pregnancy the overall size tells you nothing about each baby.

A woman expecting twins is therefore usually scanned regularly, the schedule depending on whether her twins are dichorionic or monochorionic (see Appendix). Dichorionic twin pregnancies are lower risk, so they usually get scanned at around 20 weeks, 24 weeks, 28 weeks, 32 weeks, and then every two weeks, which is the time that the growth of twins can fall off slightly compared with singletons.

Monochorionic twin pregnancies usually get fortnightly scans from 16 weeks to watch out for any signs of twin-to-twin transfusion syndrome (see Appendix, page 348). Scans usually coincide with antenatal appointments.

What if one of the babies is, for no apparent reason, growing less well in the womb? It depends on the stage of the pregnancy. Occasionally, it's a good idea to deliver both (or all) babies to give the small one a better chance. It's often said that the womb is the best incubator, but the womb becomes a hostile place for some babies, and early delivery can sometimes be better.

Early pregnancy loss

It is a sad fact of life that occasionally one or other baby does not survive the full span of the pregnancy. Some women who have early scans showing twins will lose one of the fetuses long before term. Occasionally the symptoms are like a miscarriage, with bleeding and lower abdominal cramps, but then the woman goes on feeling pregnant and her pregnancy test stays positive. This can happen if one fetus of a twin pregnancy has miscarried.

Sometimes, one baby can die without the mum having any symptoms. Although one cannot predict which women will be affected, the risk of a partial pregnancy loss is higher before twelve weeks and highest of all before eight weeks. It follows that the earlier you have a scan, the more often this phenomenon is seen. This so-called 'vanishing twin' syndrome is something which was unknown before scanning, because often the woman had no symptoms. Now it is becoming clear that it is common and may affect 20 to 30 per cent of twin pregnancies.

This kind of early pregnancy loss isn't unique to twins. There is a very high rate with singletons too. In fact, the more closely researchers look into this, the more likely it appears that many pregnancies come to grief. Unfair as it may seem, we don't know why this happens. Some experts believe that perhaps only a quarter of natural pregnancies reach full term and that 12 to 15 per cent of all live births may start off as twins.

In vanishing twin syndrome, the outlook for the surviving baby is excellent. The remaining baby will be fine, unless the miscarriage happened after the first three months of the pregnancy, which is thankfully very rare. However, if you lose one of your babies, you and your partner may have feelings you need to express to help you come to terms with the experience. You can get help from the Tamba Bereavement Support Group (page 373).

Picking up abnormalities

In many hospitals, a so-called anomaly scan is offered, usually at 20–22 weeks. An anomaly scan in twins takes twice as long as in singleton pregnancies. It can pick up various abnormalities, for instance in the heart, stomach, abdominal wall and the spine or central nervous system. However, spotting that something might be amiss is often only the first stage in diagnosing the exact problem, if any; you may need further tests. If your obstetrician is going to suggest any major intervention on the basis of USS findings, you'll almost certainly have a repeat scan to make sure any action is based on the latest and best information.

Nuchal translucency

This refers to whether or not there's a 'space', or rather a translucency filled with fluid, behind the neck of a fetus on a USS. This can be an early sign of Down's syndrome (trisomy 21) and sometimes of other disorders too, especially heart abnormalities.

It is a particularly useful sign in multiple pregnancy because so far no other effective means has been discovered of screening for Down's syndrome in twin and higher-order pregnancies. The test is offered in many centres and looks likely to become routine. It is done at 11–13 weeks, usually through the mother's abdomen, like any other USS, but to get a good picture the probe sometimes has to be placed in the vagina.

The test is said to give a result that's about 80 per cent accurate. Sometimes the result is falsely positive, in other words the baby is fine and the test was misleading. Combining it with a blood test may help make the test more specific and lower the false positive rate. Remember that nuchal translucency is just a screening method, not the final diagnosis cast in stone. If you have a positive nuchal translucency, you will be offered a further test (CVS or amniocentesis) to get a definite answer. In most cases, the results of these so-called invasive tests will still be normal, but you will be given the chance to have an anomaly scan later on anyway. In the unlikely event of an abnormality being confirmed, couples will get further advice from the hospital.

· *Antenatal Screening* ·

Having tests, and waiting for results, is worrying. On the other hand, many women find tests reassuring. There is a lot of confusion as to what antenatal tests can and cannot do and there are special problems in multiple pregnancy, so let's consider the issue as a whole.

A growing part of antenatal care is devoted to screening for a range of fetal disorders, particularly Down's syndrome and neural tube defects (NTD). NTD is the term medics give to a spectrum of central nervous system abnormalities, the best known being spina bifida and anencephaly (under-development of the whole skull). Tests can be:

- invasive (e.g. amniocentesis or CVS)
- non-invasive (e.g. USS or taking blood from the mother).

Screening in a twin or higher-order pregnancy can be difficult, either in interpreting the result (of non-invasive tests), or because an even higher level of expertise is needed to do an invasive test safely. Then, on the ethical and emotional side, what can one do about the result? If you have objections to termination under any circumstances, there is little point in having some of these antenatal tests. On the other hand, it may be that you and your obstetrician would want to be prepared for the practical and emotional challenges that can accompany the birth of special needs babies. You will have your own view, shaped by your values, beliefs and social circumstances.

Twin pregnancies where only one baby is affected present a further dilemma. It is now possible in some circumstances selectively to terminate a multiple pregnancy (this topic is covered in the Appendix), a decision which is a huge responsibility for any couple facing this situation. It is bad enough to lose and grieve for a singleton, but psychologists have found that mourning for one baby while simultaneously caring for another of the same age can create conflict. On the other hand, multiples can be challenging enough to parent when healthy, let alone when one of them is severely disabled.

Then there are the general cautions which ought to be (but are not always) given with all antenatal screening. Results are rarely 100 per cent positive or negative and they can occasionally mislead. Many screening tests only give the probability of a baby being affected and the figures are not always easy to understand. If the result is greater than one in 250 (say it's one in 150), the test is usually said to be positive. If the result is smaller than one in 250 (say one in 400), it's said to be negative (yes, that is the right way round).

An added complication is that, even when you have a firm diagnosis, from a test like CVS for example, it still does not tell you how seriously affected this particular baby is likely to be. As an example, anencephaly is fairly straightforward because it's usually lethal, but a child who has Down's syndrome can be very happy and affectionate, and fulfilling to parent. Need I point out that not every so-called normal child is all of those things?

All this may sound depressing, but pregnant women and the professionals caring for them should consider these issues in advance, not after the lab sends a positive result. In fact, a negative (that is, normal) result is far and away the likeliest outcome, and receiving it can be very reassuring. But realism demands a note of caution: screening doesn't tell you absolutely everything is OK. In the last analysis, life and creating life are still something of a gamble. There is no such thing as a guarantee of a perfect baby.

> *When I was pregnant, my partner and I sought out hard-and-fast answers. We were desperate to be sure our baby would be 100 per cent OK. But I soon worked it out: if it's a guarantee you're after, don't have a family – buy a toaster.*

You won't need much luck, because over 98 per cent of babies overall are born completely healthy. Chances are you won't have to face any of these dilemmas. However, it is important to know, before you have any tests, the route you could be taking. Your obstetrician, GP or midwife can give you information about testing, though ultimately you and your partner have to make up your own minds.

Your worries

With twins or higher multiples, you may be more worried than with a singleton pregnancy. After all, aren't two or more healthy babies a lot to ask for? But in fact abnormalities are not that much more common with multiples than with single babies. Down's syndrome, for instance, is no more likely, as long as you allow for the fact that mothers of twins tend to be slightly older. A few identical twins seem to run a slightly higher risk of some conditions, mostly abnormalities of the midline body organs, but these are really extremely rare. Cerebral palsy is estimated to be more common in multiples, though this may be because more small, vulnerable babies are surviving.

Some anxiety is part and parcel of pregnancy (and parenting). It would be unusual to find an expectant mother who didn't have any concerns about her unborn babies. Of course, if worry begins to take over and interfere with your ability to enjoy life or to look forward to your babies, you need to talk things over with someone you trust, like your midwife or doctor. You can also call Tamba Twinline.

· *Non-invasive Tests* ·

Nuchal translucency and anomaly scans were both covered earlier, in the section on ultrasound scans. The other common non-invasive tests are AFP and the so-called triple test.

Alphafetoprotein (AFP)

This is a blood test that you can have at around 16 weeks of pregnancy. It screens for spina bifida and other NTDs. AFP is a protein made by the baby's liver, and a certain amount spills over into the mother's bloodstream, hence its usefulness. A high AFP level may indicate a higher risk of spina bifida and NTDs, but twinning also raises AFP because there are two babies making the protein. So, whilst a very high level can be helpful, on the whole AFP levels are misleading with multiples and of course tell you nothing about the health of each individual baby.

Some women happen to have an AFP test before their first scan and therefore before they know they are having twins, so they may be told that their result is 'too high' and suffer all the anxiety that this entails. However, once the scan confirms twins, you can usually be reassured.

Double test and triple test

These are two very popular blood tests, also known as the Bart's test and Leeds test. You may know about them because they are widely offered to women expecting single-tons. Unfortunately they are not helpful with multiples. Work is now being carried out to see whether the tests can be applied to twins and higher multiples (for instance by applying a mathematical correction factor to the result), but it will probably be some time before these tests can be considered reliable in such cases.

· Invasive Tests ·

The two main invasive tests are amniocentesis and CVS (chorionic villus sampling), and their main use is in giving an exact diagnosis. For a pregnant woman, the prospect of an invasive test can be more scary than any fear of needles. She is usually worried about the small risk of miscarriage from the test, especially if she is an older mother. The snag is that it is mainly more mature women who benefit most from these tests.

Amniocentesis

This involves taking a sample of the amniotic fluid around each baby. It also collects a few of the cells floating free in the fluid and therefore gives information about chromosome abnormalities, such as Down's syndrome, which are more common in older mothers. You may be offered the test if you are over 38 or 40 years old, or have had a screening test which suggests amniocentesis might be a good idea.

Amniocentesis is done in the second three months of pregnancy, usually at about 16 weeks or more. (Technically, it can be done earlier, but this sometimes makes it more risky.) Because cells usually have to be grown in the laboratory to yield a result, you may have to wait till nearly 20 weeks before you know the outcome of the test. Newer lab techniques can give a result within 48 hours of amniocentesis, but you may have to pay for the sample to be sent to a private lab.

The test is done through the abdomen (using local anaesthetic), with a fine needle for each baby, and under ultrasound control to avoid damaging the fetuses or their placentas. To make sure that fluid from around both babies is sampled, dye can be injected into one of the amniotic cavities during the test.

The risk of miscarriage from amniocentesis is slightly under 1 per cent. The percentage may be lower if the procedure is carried out using only one needle, which goes through the fetal membranes to sample both sacs. Infection can also be a complication, but it's rare. The most common after-effect is some cramping discomfort for the woman. Whether one or two needles are used, it is technically difficult to do with twins and higher multiples, so you usually need to be referred to a specialist fetal medicine centre.

Chorionic villus sampling (CVS)

Like amniocentesis, CVS gives information about a baby's chromosomes, but this test samples cells directly from the chorionic villi, which are fragments of the placenta.

CVS is done with a needle through the abdomen or sometimes via the cervix; with multiples it may be done through both. Again, a little local anaesthetic is used and ultrasound control is essential.

The big plus of CVS is that it gives results sooner than amniocentesis, first because it is done earlier, at around 11–13 weeks, and second because cells don't have to be grown in the lab before being examined. On the minus side, dye cannot be injected during the CVS test. So if the tests yield two lots of genetically identical tissue, it may be impossible to know whether material from both babies has been sampled, or whether you have identical twins.

The risk of miscarriage from CVS is also around 1 per cent. There's the additional risk of abnormalities of the fingers or toes if the test is done before 10 weeks. For this reason, it is usually done at 11 weeks at the earliest. CVS demands skill and experience in any pregnancy, but especially when carried out with multiples, which is why you may need to go to a specialist fetal medicine centre.

· *Caring for Yourself during Pregnancy* ·

Because having multiples puts extra demands on your body and may cause more minor aches and symptoms in pregnancy, it is worth taking good care of yourself – and thereby of your babies too. The best news of all is that the steps you take while pregnant can be of lasting benefit to your babies' health, and yours.

Smoking

If you or your partner smoke, this is an excellent time to stop for good. I know this is going to sound like a lecture, and you know it's going to be a lecture, because at heart we all realise there's nothing good to say about cigarette smoke. It contains carbon monoxide, which robs the body of oxygen, as well as a cocktail of toxic chemicals including cancer-causing substances, and nicotine to keep you hooked. My excuse for raising the issue here is that smoking is especially harmful in twin and higher multiple pregnancies.

Firstly, miscarriage is more common in women who smoke, or are passive smokers. Smoking, even passively, is also strongly linked with the birth of premature, low-birth-weight, sicklier babies. Research from Denmark confirms that the harmful effects are greater for twins than for singletons, a vital point since twins are already prone to being premature and vulnerable.

Secondly, the effects of smoking linger. Babies born to smokers have a higher risk of cot death (sudden infant death syndrome or SIDS), allergies, asthma, chest infections and glue ear.

Nicotine replacement treatment can be a big help in giving up, though it's not usually advised during pregnancy. However, there are other methods than can help, so if you smoke or live with someone who does, talk to your doctor or midwife early on.

Food and drink

The general recommendations for pregnant women are covered in many other books and leaflets, so this section focuses mainly on the special needs of those expecting twins or more.

Your aim is a balanced diet that is enough to nourish you and your babies. However overweight you are to begin with, don't try to lose any weight during your pregnancy. You must gain weight in pregnancy, so dieting in any form has to wait. For now, what you must do is eat well and often, to establish early weight gain. Morning sickness can be a problem, but eating smaller portions more often should do it.

During this pregnancy, you can assume that you need 50 per cent to 100 per cent more of important nutrients like iron, calcium, folic acid and vitamin B12. An important exception is vitamin A, which could be harmful to the fetus if taken in excess. This is the main reason why pregnant women should avoid eating liver or taking cod-liver oil.

If you eat well and have no complications or other medical

conditions, you are unlikely to need vitamin tablets, but this is a controversial area. Some nutritionists believe that the usual recommended daily allowances may be enough to stave off the typical deficiency diseases, like scurvy or pellagra, yet be insufficient for optimum health. If you want to take vitamins while pregnant, check first with your midwife, doctor or pharmacist. Avoid taking any extra vitamin A in tablet form. However, it's safe and even healthy to have carrots, swede, apricots and other foods which are rich in beta-carotene, the forerunner of vitamin A.

All women who are planning to conceive, or are in the first 12 weeks of pregnancy, should take a daily folic acid supplement of 400 microgrammes (0.4 mg) to lower the risk of spina bifida and other NTDs. You also need to eat foods rich in folate, like leafy green vegetables, black-eyed peas and folate-enriched bread.

Achieving a balanced diet means eating several portions a day from each of these food groups:

- Cereals, breads, rice and pasta – for carbohydrates (energy), fibre, protein and vitamins. Choose wholemeal and wholegrain products if possible, and avoid too many refined carbohydrates (cakes, biscuits, etc.).
- Fruit, vegetables and salads – for vitamins (especially folate and vitamin C), fibre and minerals. Make sure all salads are washed well – there is a risk of toxoplasmosis from soil – and cook vegetables lightly to preserve vitamins.
- Fish, meat, poultry, eggs and pulses – for protein, iron and vitamin B12. Avoid undercooked meat (because of the risk of toxoplasmosis) and undercooked poultry (because of the risk of salmonella and campylobacter). Eggs should be cooked until the yolk goes hard (to guard against salmonella). If you are a vegetarian, eat plenty of pulses and use yeast extracts, which are rich in B12. It's best to avoid nuts if there's a strong family history of allergies.

● Milk, cheese and other dairy products – for calcium and protein. On average, a woman pregnant with twins or more needs five daily servings to ensure she gets enough calcium. One serving is a yoghurt, a glass of milk, or about 30 grams (1 oz) of cheese. Low-fat milks contain as much calcium as full-fat. Pilchards, sardines and tinned salmon (with the small bones) are also rich in calcium.

Pregnant women are more at risk from bacteria called listeria and should avoid soft ripened cheeses (like Brie), blue-veined cheeses, pâté of all kinds and cook-chilled foods (unless these are properly heated through).

You also need plenty of fluids, by which I mean non-alcoholic beverages like water and fruit juices. A frequent piece of advice to pregnant women is to avoid all alcoholic drinks. However, small amounts can be safe, as long as it's just the very occasional drink. There's no need to deprive yourself of the odd celebratory glass, for instance. It should go without saying, however, that illicit or 'street' drugs are a particularly bad idea in pregnancy.

Rest and exercise

Getting enough rest is an important part of pregnancy. Besides, you are going to be very busy for the next few years. Many pregnant women feel energetic, and others less so. There are no hard-and-fast rules here, because multiple pregnancies tend to vary far more than do singleton pregnancies. Some women carrying twins have been known to continue with athletic feats, while a few are scarcely able to drag themselves around the shops.

As a rule, pelvic-floor exercises are essential, and swimming is almost always useful – even if you cannot swim, you will feel nicely buoyant in the water.

What of sport and other exercises? Of course exercise is

good for health, and it's unnecessary to recline for weeks on end like a Victorian heroine with an attack of the vapours. However, you should know that vigorous or sustained exercise can rob the uterus of blood, and could even trigger contractions. For the sake of your babies, it's unwise to take up a new sport unless it's a gentle pursuit. Any exercise that could inflict a direct blow to your growing bump is out, especially towards the end of your pregnancy. The heat generated by exercise can be important too. For the sake of your babies, your body temperature should not rise too high, especially in early pregnancy. Avoid exercising in hot weather, or at high altitude, which puts extra strain on the circulation.

As a rule, you can go on doing your usual exercises, except for such things as endurance activities, contact sports and scuba diving, but check with your midwife or doctor if in doubt.

Your own health and safety are also concerns. A woman's centre of gravity changes in pregnancy as her abdomen grows. Moreover, her joints and ligaments become softer, thanks to a pregnancy hormone called relaxin. So, whatever you do, be sure to pace yourself and listen to your body. Stop if you get discomfort, ask for advice when you're unsure, and let your babies be your guide. It is sometimes said that if your babies kick mainly at night, you are not getting enough rest in the day. There is some logic in this adage, since womb space is restricted and there is obviously less room for kicking about when your own muscles are in action all the time.

As your pregnancy advances, you should reduce your activities, and make a point of getting a nap every afternoon. With a big bump to sustain, you will not be able to carry on doing it all, whether at home or at work (or both). This applies especially if you already have one or more children clamouring for attention.

Towards the end of my twin pregnancy, Larissa had her second birthday. When she wanted a cuddle, she had to climb up for it. I learned that I really couldn't pick her up any more, and I stopped trying. My rule had to be: if she's conscious, don't lift her!

Sometimes eating well, scaling down your activities, and perhaps getting help with chores is not enough, and you may be advised to take a proper rest. The more babies you are carrying, the more likely you are to have to go into hospital before the due date. The National Study of Triplets and Higher Order Births showed that 95 per cent of women expecting triplets (and all those with quads) were admitted to hospital at least once during their pregnancy. This may be changing. In 1998, Tamba carried out a huge survey into maternity services, getting replies from nearly 600 women from all over the UK, all of whom had delivered twins or triplets in 1997. Some 32 per cent of twin mums and 65 per cent of triplet mums had been admitted to hospital for rest before delivery, typically for raised blood pressure or pre-eclampsia.

It was once thought that rest, especially in bed, was in itself beneficial in pregnancy, but this does not seem to be the case. However, rest in hospital is still helpful for some complications and of course also puts you and your babies where the neonatal facilities are. Bed rest does seem to increase blood flow to the placenta, and can reduce the weight on the cervix, but it has not been shown to reduce the risk of premature labour; nor does it live up to all the claims made for it in the past. Languishing in bed also carries hazards, such as the risk of deep-vein thrombosis (a known complication of pregnancy, especially multiple pregnancy), and muscle wasting from lack of use.

Fortunately, nowadays bed rest is prescribed not so much for its own sake but to enable various complications to be treated or anticipated, for instance by a short period of monitoring in hospital.

Some women are relieved to be in hospital, with its high-tech facilities, and to be away from the demands of a busy home or workplace. But being away from home has obvious drawbacks: strange surroundings, noise, sleep deprivation, lack of privacy – and hospital food. This is often the subject of jokes, but it's no laughing matter. In many cases hospital fare is barely adequate for women expecting singletons, let alone those with multiples.

You are more likely to agree to go into hospital if there is a good reason, so ask your doctor rather than accepting a stay unquestioningly, or refusing flatly. If you live nearby, you may find that you and your obstetrician can reach a compromise which enables you to rest at home. But note that rest really does mean rest, with someone else looking after the home and any younger children. It does not mean sitting with your feet up for 10 minutes before leaping up to do the laundry, get the meals, and so on.

When my wife went into hospital at 33 weeks for pre-eclampsia, a friend had Amy, then aged two, for most of the day. My boss agreed that I could leave work early to look after her from about 4 p.m. I never thought we'd cope, but we did superbly even if I say so myself. And it was worth it because the twins were born at 35 weeks and all was well.

Sex

This can be a problem during pregnancy for several reasons. You may be tired or uncomfortable, or perhaps you've just gone off the idea, especially if you are having a lot of symptoms or find it hard to adapt to your impending role as a mother (as tends to be the case in a first pregnancy). Alternatively, your partner may have gone off it: while some men find the pregnant shape appealing, others do not. Perhaps you or your partner are afraid of hurting the babies; you may have noticed that they often kick a lot more after intercourse.

If you do feel like it, there is no reason why you should not have intercourse during your multiple pregnancy, provided you have no complications, such as premature contractions or vaginal bleeding, and have not been told by your doctor to abstain. Obstetricians vary a bit as to what they consider safe in multiple pregnancies, and each pregnancy is different too. If in doubt, check.

That said, your most taxing problem is one of logistics. As the weeks go by, you will have to use your imagination to get close to each other. You may find you prefer to give up on penetrative sex and use other means to pleasure each other.

· *Coping with Common Symptoms* ·

Indigestion and nausea

'Morning' sickness and indigestion or heartburn tend to be worse during a multiple pregnancy, especially when the babies are growing well. These symptoms are caused by the enlarging bump as well as hormones. Progesterone, for example, relaxes the muscle at the entrance to the stomach, letting stomach acid flow back up the gullet and cause the searing sensation of heartburn.

You can minimise both heartburn and nausea by:

- avoiding fatty or spicy foods, or anything which you know from experience can upset your stomach
- eating frequent small snacks of carbohydrate – dry biscuits, toast, etc.
- drinking milk or taking mild antacids – ask your midwife or

chemist; if you need anything on prescription, remember that you are exempt from NHS prescription charges during pregnancy

- avoiding heavy meals just before bedtime
- sleeping with two or more pillows, so that your head is higher than your stomach
- avoiding tight clothes – be honest when your jeans no longer fit! When you are pregnant with twins, you may eventually find you even get too large for some maternity clothes.

If you can't keep food down, tell your doctor. Some anti-sickness tablets can help in pregnancy, but it is best to check first.

Constipation

The hormone progesterone tends to relax the gut and make bowel action sluggish.

You can help avoid constipation by:

- eating plenty of fibre-rich foods
- taking regular exercise, even if it is only a daily walk.

Don't take laxatives unless your doctor or midwife approves. They can be harmful in pregnancy.

Piles (haemorrhoids)

Increased pressure inside the abdomen in the latter half of pregnancy makes piles more common, especially with twins, but constipation at any time can also bring them on.

Typical symptoms are itching and a painful swelling near the back passage (anus). If you have any bleeding, see your doctor; it may or may not be piles.

- Watch your diet to keep your bowels regular.
- Try not to strain or sit on the toilet for long periods of time.
- When you need to go, go then. Don't put it off till later. Delay makes motions harder.
- Use soft toilet paper. If you already have itching or a lump, wash often. Wet wipes kept in your handbag are useful when out and about.
- Check with your doctor or chemist before using any of the available over-the-counter remedies for haemorrhoids.

Backache

Low back pain is common in twin pregnancy, first because the extra load puts the spine under greater mechanical strain, and second because the abdominal muscles are more stretched and cannot do their bit to stabilise the spine. Also, the hormone relaxin, which softens ligaments in the spine and elsewhere in preparation for labour, makes minor aches and injuries more likely.

- Try to keep your spine straight. Avoid standing with the small of the back fully curved in the typical pregnant posture. Instead, tuck your buttocks in and tilt the front of your pelvis up.
- Wearing flattish shoes is better for your posture.
- Don't bend your back when bending forwards. (In any case, you will eventually be unable to.) Bend at the knees instead when picking anything off the floor. Better still, go down on one knee.
- Take care when getting into and out of bed, especially in late pregnancy. Roll on to your side first then put your feet on the floor before sitting up.
- Avoid press-ups, sit-ups and heavy lifting. Don't rearrange furniture unaided and carry your toddler only when absolutely necessary.

- Go swimming – it is one of the things you can often enjoy until late in pregnancy, if you can find a large enough swimsuit. Some women who are pregnant with twins find they outgrow many maternity swimsuits, so alterations may be needed.
- Specific back exercises can both prevent and relieve backache, for instance getting on all fours and alternately arching your back and letting it sag. Your antenatal teacher can tell you about others.
- When your back hurts, a warm bath (not hot), a gentle massage from your partner and the odd paracetamol can all help. Avoid other drugs unless you've checked with your doctor or pharmacist.

Varicose veins

Because of your growing bump and your hormonal changes, prominent or bulging leg veins, with or without aching, are common in pregnancy. You won't necessarily get varicose veins; family history is a factor too.

- When sitting, keep your feet up on a stool or coffee table rather than dangling down.
- Don't stand for long periods of time. If you must, keep moving your legs.
- Walking is a good form of exercise and will keep blood flowing rather than stagnating in your leg veins.
- Maternity support tights help.

Insomnia

During the last few weeks of pregnancy, as your bump becomes increasingly large and exciting thoughts go whizzing round your head, sleeplessness can be a real nuisance.

- Wind down to bedtime with a restful routine. Avoid coffee, tea and caffeinated soft drinks in the evening.
- Make yourself as comfortable as you can. Lying on your back can make you feel faint because the womb will press on your major blood vessels. So try lying on your side with the help of a pillow or two to support your abdomen.
- Use the relaxation technique you learned in antenatal classes.
- If you are worried about something, bring the issue out into the open and discuss it with your partner, or jot down the questions you'd like to ask your midwife when you next see her.

Skin changes

Stretch marks are common after a twin pregnancy, but they are not inevitable and many women don't get them. However, in the last month or two, itchy skin on the lower abdomen or the back bothers many pregnant women. This is thought to be caused by dryness and stretching of the skin.

- Avoid scratching if possible, because it releases the chemical histamine into the skin, which makes itching worse.
- Keep your skin smooth with bath oils and body lotions, preferably unperfumed. The worst areas may respond to Vaseline or calamine lotion.
- Baths should be warm rather than hot.
- If you get itching all over the body or in unusual places (for instance, on your hands and feet), contact your doctor, especially if you also have dark urine or pale stools. You may have cholestasis of pregnancy. I only mention this rare condition in case you don't come across it anywhere else. It is no more common in twin pregnancy but needs to be recognised promptly as it can cause stillbirth. The usual

treatment is close monitoring of the mother combined with early delivery of the babies.

Swollen hands and feet

Mild swelling of the feet, and to some extent the fingers, is not unusual, especially on a hot day in the later stages of pregnancy. However, you should always bring it to the notice of your midwife or doctor just in case it is a sign of pre-eclampsia.

As long as all's well, just try to make things easier for yourself, and:

- wear comfortable shoes
- rest with your feet up when possible
- avoid standing unnecessarily
- wear maternity support tights
- remove rings before your fingers get too podgy.

· *Preparing Yourself for Twins or More* ·

As you approach the big day, emotional preparation can be as important as taking physical care of yourself. By now, you and your nearest and dearest may feel well adjusted to the idea of having more than one baby, but unless there are twins in your family or immediate circle of friends, you cannot appreciate all the implications. As several nurses and midwives have themselves found out, you don't know what it is like to have multiple babies until you experience it at first hand.

Attend antenatal and parentcraft classes in good time. Multiples tend to arrive early and often with little warning. Even if yours stay the course, you may not feel up to travelling to and from the hospital in the last few weeks. If you try to complete antenatal classes at least a month ahead of women expecting singletons, you probably won't miss much.

Few hospitals have any antenatal teaching aimed at women expecting multiples, though the number is increasing. Tamba's maternity services survey found that 21 per cent of mothers attended one or more specific antenatal sessions for multiples, and 93 per cent found them helpful. Even if you are a second- or third-time mother, do go to any special sessions for prospective parents of twins. The benefits are palpable. Midwifery researcher Debbie Sen found that extra antenatal preparation tailored to twin pregnancies helped mums to cope better after the birth, and to feel more positive about parenting.

The content of ordinary antenatal and parentcraft classes is geared exclusively towards single births. This makes it very hard for expectant mothers to get appropriate information. But don't hesitate to speak up and ask whether particular aspects mentioned will apply to you.

If you live within striking distance of London, you may like to attend one of the MBF's prenatal evening meetings for prospective parents (and grandparents) of multiples; contact the MBF direct.

Make sure you visit the Special Care Baby Unit (SCBU) on the tour of your own hospital, as your babies have a higher chance of spending time there. In Tamba's maternity survey, 39 per cent of mums with a baby in Special Care hadn't seen the unit in advance.

Find out too about what your hospital offers in the way of pain relief (in the next chapter there is more on this and other aspects of labour, including caesareans). When you are ready, start making a birth plan, but try to be flexible.

You may like to start interacting with your babies by stroking your bump, or talking or singing. Babies can feel, hear, and even see long before birth. In the last few months of pregnancy, they see well enough to distinguish light from dark. A baby responds to a gentle prod at five months and can react to noise from around 16 weeks, swaying to the sound of his mother's voice. A baby remembers too. He can learn a tune that is played repeatedly before birth, and recognise it after he is born. At birth, babies show a preference for their mother's voice, suggesting that useful skills are learnt while still in the womb (interestingly, they even get used to the foods Mum normally eats, as traces of it appear in amniotic fluid). This is important in terms of each baby's attachment to you, and you can help this along.

There's now good evidence that a baby's prenatal environment affects later development. How much a fetus can feel or even think is a thorny issue, but it is clear that women who are seriously stressed tend to have babies who become hyperactive. This is not necessarily cause-and-effect, but it may be: stress hormones can be shown to reduce blood flow in the placenta. Unfortunately, you cannot become placid on demand, though you can try to unwind with relaxation techniques. The ancient Chinese probably knew this. As far back as 1000 BC, there were pregnancy clinics developed to keep mothers calm before the birth.

Read the next few chapters and think ahead about practical matters. Will you want to breast-feed? How will you manage in the first few days at home? Where will the babies sleep? Get a minimum of baby equipment organised. Many mothers-to-be are superstitious, and there could also be financial reasons not to stock up on everything in advance, but you will need some items from the earliest days. You may be able to borrow enough from friends.

It helps a lot to meet others in your area who already have twins or who are expecting them. Contact Tamba direct if the hospital cannot put you in touch with your local group. Twins' clubs can help you make friends and find out more about the practicalities of caring for twins. You will also get the chance to borrow books and perhaps to see Tamba's pregnancy and birth video, *Expecting More than One* (you may prefer to buy this). Often the clubs are also excellent sources of good second-hand baby equipment.

Try to prepare your family for the big event. Seeing the scan (or a photo of it) and attending clinic appointments can help bring the reality home to your partner, but it can also create worries which need to be talked through. Debbie Sen's research on antenatal preparation aimed specially at twins underlines this. She found that dads who attended appointments and classes were better prepared and more involved in parenting, and this had a positive effect on the couple's relationship.

Some men aren't good at expressing their emotions, but your partner may be just as concerned as you are about the health of your babies. He may have his own anxieties too. As a father of twins, his role is likely to be more hands-on. How will he cope with his job as well as lending you practical help? Can he take leave from work? Will he now have to work harder to make up for the loss of your income?

If the pregnancy was unplanned, how will you both embrace your new status as parents – not just of one baby, but of two or more? It can be double the shock if you hadn't intended to conceive yet (or at all). As well as discussing matters together, you may both benefit from talking things over with someone outside the family: a GP, midwife, psychologist (ask your GP), or stress counsellor at work.

Grandparents may need educating too. The older generation can be unduly pessimistic about twins because the outlook was less good in their day. On the other hand, grandparents sometimes have unrealistic notions about how wonderful twins, triplets or more can be. Understandably, they'll want to brag, but they also need to appreciate that you will need help in caring for two or more little individuals. A fortunate few may find a grandparent is able to help with the cost of an au pair, maternity nurse or mother's help. Some women opt for a doula, a mother or sister substitute who can support you before and after the birth.

The birth of two or more siblings at once is bound to be a challenging time for any children you already have. Give your older child as much time and attention as you can now, and work out what you will do when you go into hospital. You will find lots more ideas on relationships in Chapter 9.

Make plans for your own job. Will you return to work after the birth? You cannot know now how you will feel – even if you're fairly sure you are leaving for good, it is sometimes best to tell your employer that you are undecided. Once a permanent replacement is ensconced in your office, it could be impossible to return.

Perhaps you are contemplating a change, to a part-time job or to hours that fit in better with a double dose of parenting. Employers now have a legal duty to consider requests for flexible working from parents of children under six years old.

Your employer must give you time off work to attend for antenatal care, which generally means antenatal classes too. However, whatever you can do to minimise the impact on your work could be appreciated. Can you make up the work some other time?

If this is your first pregnancy, you may want to press on with work until you drop (or your twins do). Many women prefer to take their paid maternity leave after the birth rather than before, but this is unrealistic with a multiple pregnancy. Most experts suggest that you stop working a bit sooner if you are expecting twins or more. Other things being equal, it is reasonable to go on maternity leave from the twenty-ninth week of pregnancy until the babies are six months old – at least. Statutory maternity pay is paid for up to 26 weeks, and you may also qualify for up to 26 weeks of additional maternity leave. Your partner is now also entitled to two weeks' paid paternity leave. You can find out about your entitlements from antenatal clinics and the DSS.

It all depends on how your pregnancy is going – multiple pregnancies vary a lot. So do jobs. Health and Safety at Work regulations require employers to take account of particular risks to pregnant employees and new mothers. If risks cannot be avoided by other means, working hours or conditions have to change. Otherwise you must have paid leave for as long as necessary to protect your health and that of your babies. You can get more information from the Health and Safety Executive.

Whatever your job, severe morning sickness may lead you to want a later start to your working day. Even a sedentary job can make you very tired. A lunchtime or early afternoon rest, taken lying down, helps fight fatigue and may also improve placental blood flow. Don't be shy about asking: you're responsible for the next generation. Besides, employers are now obliged to provide rest facilities for pregnant (or breast-feeding) workers.

The commute can become difficult. As many heavily pregnant women discover, you can practically give birth on a crowded train before anyone bats an eyelid, let alone does anything useful like give up their seat. The solution may be a parking space at work, so that you can drive.

Work itself may be more taxing. Many pregnant women say their brains turn to mush, making simple tasks much harder. This isn't an illusion: MRI scans show that a woman's brain actually shrinks during pregnancy, but it seems to recover afterwards. Nobody knows whether the effect is any worse with twin or triplet pregnancies.

Start thinking of names and draw up a short (or long?) list of your favourites for both boys and girls, unless you already know which you are expecting. This may save you from making hasty decisions after the birth, or calling your babies 'Pink Blanket' and 'White Blanket' for three days until you and your partner agree.

A child's name is an integral part of his individuality and personality and choosing names for multiples, while double or treble the fun, needs care. Names like Kirsten and Christine which sound very similar will be difficult. Try also to avoid rhyming names (Jenny and Penny), and two or more names with the same initial (Thomas and Theresa may find it hard at the same school). Thinking of how the names sound when abbreviated will help you steer clear of John and Malcolm, or Philip and William.

Matching names (Jade and Amber, Holly and Ivy) sound witty at the time, but your children may not share the joke. Names which are very different in length (like Christopher and Luke) can seem a good idea, but sometimes pose problems when the children are learning to write.

Consider too what the names sound like together. When talking about your children to someone who doesn't know them, Lily and Mary may be mistaken for the single name Lilian Mary. (Reversing the order won't help, because Mary and Lily sounds like Marian Lily.)

You may like to name your twins or triplets in reverse alphabetical order, so that the first-born is called Natasha and the second-born Andrew. Then at least Andrew will come first in something, which could count for a lot in later childhood.

Some families even use different surnames for their twins, one from the mother and the other from the father. This could work if the mother uses her maiden name anyway.

Take old wives' tales with a pinch of salt, whether they are about childbirth in general or multiples in particular. You may have heard that labour is the most painful experience on earth (not true), or that the girl of a boy-girl pair of twins is always sterile (only in cattle). Discount these and other myths that could affect your peace of mind.

You are bound to have a few questions, worries or doubts, but the more unresolved problems you have, the less you will enjoy your pregnancy. Although clinics and surgeries are busy places, always consult your doctor or midwife if you have medical queries. Medics tend to shy away from patients with long written lists (said to be a sure sign of a hypochondriac!), so be assertive if necessary. And prioritise. Don't leave your most burning question till last, as doctors can get called away.

If the person you ask can't answer all your questions, try a different member of the team, or call Tamba Twinline. If any of the professionals you meet needs more information on multiples, you can put them in touch with Tamba or MBF, each of which has a role in educating professionals.

Lastly, put yourself first. Social and psychological support antenatally can help avert problems and even postnatal depression. You should still get continuity of antenatal care even when you are expecting multiples. Tamba's maternity services survey showed that two-thirds of the mothers usually saw the same doctor at each hospital visit. If you need to see a social worker too, just ask. It can make all the difference. Talking to your health visitor before the birth is useful too.

Some women and their partners find it hard to get used to their new role as parents of twins. It's worth spending time together as a couple and building on the relationship before the babies arrive. Try to enjoy the pregnancy as much as you can. It is an exciting time, and chances are you won't have multiples again!

Adjusting can take time. Maybe you won't entirely adjust until after the event. A few mothers resent twins, and grieve for the cosy one-to-one relationship they might have had with a single baby.

I only had six weeks at home with my first son, so I was going to take much longer off work after my second baby and really get to know him or her. I was also determined to breast-feed for longer. But my plans were completely shot by the fact that the second baby was not one but two. I now think they are the best thing that ever happened to me. But it was months before I got used to the idea of them being twins.

Once they get over this, many delights are in store.

Chapter Three

THE BIG DAY: LABOUR AND BIRTH

When my waters broke at 9 p.m., I knew there was no going back. Within 20 minutes my husband had rushed me to the labour ward. We'd forgotten my hospital bag, but you can't have everything.

Unless your hospital makes special provision for women expecting more than one, some of what you are told about labour and birth in antenatal classes won't apply to you. First, some reassuring facts:

- Labour with twins is not twice as painful or twice as long as with singletons. It can even be less uncomfortable because the babies tend to be a bit smaller.
- No matter how many babies there are in there, the cervix needs to dilate fully only once for them to get out, so there's just one first stage of labour.
- Although birth is more hazardous for twins and triplets, the outlook is improving all the time.

It's natural to be concerned about how labour will be for you and your babies. While you should not underestimate the potential difficulties, it helps not to be fearful. This is where being informed comes in. If anything worries you, ask your doctor or midwife early on. The answer may put your mind at rest.

In general, the more relaxed you are, the better the birth will be. Emotions such as fear and anxiety are linked with raised levels of hormones like adrenalin, which makes muscles tense up. Midwives even say that a tense jaw during labour makes for an unyielding perineum. You may well find that on the day you will be happier and calmer than you anticipated. Women tend to rise to the occasion of birth, and again it could be partly hormonal. Certainly the pregnancy hormone pregnanolone has been dubbed a natural tranquilliser.

· *Premature Labour* ·

You need to know about premature labour and how to recognise it because, unlike trains, twins and higher multiples tend to arrive ahead of schedule. As compared with singletons, premature (pre-term) birth is actually six times more common in twins, and about 11 times more common in triplets. Although all the vital organs form in the first three months of pregnancy, babies actually grow at their fastest rate in the last three months. This brings home just how important prematurity can be. One piece of good news: at the same stage of pregnancy, twins tend to be more developed than single babies. So please don't panic, especially when it comes to minor degrees of prematurity.

Normally 'full term' for twins is 37 weeks, while triplets often arrive at 34 weeks and quads at 32 weeks, as mentioned in the last chapter. Anything earlier than this is considered premature, but obviously there are differences of degree. Twins born a few days short of 37 weeks don't face the same dangers as those born at 28 weeks.

- About 30 per cent of twins are pre-term, while the figure for singletons is only 10 per cent.
- About 30 per cent of triplets are born before 32 weeks and 10 per cent are born before 28 weeks.

- For quads, there is less information available, but nearly half deliver before 32 weeks, and 25 per cent before 28 weeks.

Which babies arrive early?

Premature labour is more common in identical (MZ) twins, especially if there is only one chorionic membrane and if they are boys. The reason is not clear, but funnily enough male singletons are also more likely to deliver early.

If you are expecting twins in your first pregnancy, you are more likely to go into labour prematurely than if this is your second or subsequent pregnancy.

What causes prematurity?

During a multiple pregnancy, there are often more contractions of the Braxton-Hicks type. These are low-strength contractions which are commonly described as the womb 'getting into training'. It is not surprising that in multiple pregnancy the muscle of the uterus is a bit more taut and irritable, as it were – after all, it has more to contend with.

In themselves, Braxton-Hicks contractions don't spell premature labour, though they can precede it. Labour involves not just uterine contractions, but the cervix changing, softening and beginning to dilate.

In a typical normal labour, hormones called prostaglandins make the cervix ripen, rather like a soft fruit. Several other hormones, especially oestrogen and oxytocin, play a role too. Oestrogen levels rise at the end of pregnancy and trigger more prostaglandin release from the lining of the uterus. Meanwhile, the woman's pituitary gland produces more oxytocin to make the uterus contract (the synthetic version, Syntocinon, is sometimes given by injection during labour to speed it up). The hormone relaxin probably has a part too, and so does the natural ageing of the placenta as it reaches the end of its useful life.

What sparks off the process? It's not just the womb being stretched to capacity. If it were, more twins would be born at 28–30 weeks, when the size of the uterus is like that of a singleton at term. Perhaps surprisingly, the timing of a normal labour has a lot to do with the babies. It's a fetus's own hormones from his adrenal glands (near the kidneys) that kick off the whole process.

Nobody knows what starts premature labour. Perhaps with multiples the fetal membranes (the chorion and amnion) simply produce more prostaglandins, which stimulate the womb to contract. Or maybe the uterus is more sensitive to oxytocin. Research shows that infection is a cause of pre-term labour in about a third of singletons born too soon, and this might work by producing enzymes in the chorion and amnion. It's not certain how relevant this is to twins, though.

A lax cervix is a cause too sometimes. Smoking is also linked with premature (prem) labour, for reasons which are still unknown.

There is a well-known link between poor growth in the womb and premature labour. How it works isn't obvious, but it makes perfect sense. If the environment's inhospitable, then it's not in a baby's best interests to stay there. There's some evidence that rest and good nutrition can help prevent labour from starting too soon, but once it has started there is a limit to what can be done.

Symptoms of premature labour

Whatever actually starts things off, it is vital to be aware of the possible symptoms. You owe it to your babies to know the warning signs and what action to take. This bit is not meant to alarm either you or your partner, but to give you the information everyone pregnant with multiples needs. As in any labour, you may start getting:

- regular contractions (every 10 to 15 minutes)
- pain in the lower belly, pelvis or back
- an unusually heavy feeling in the pelvis
- blood or mucus from the vagina (either of which can indicate changes in the cervix)
- clear fluid from the vagina (this usually indicates ruptured membranes).

Contact the labour ward if you have any of these symptoms. If you are not sure of the significance of your symptoms, check with the labour ward anyway. You can ignore reassuring noises from friends who have singletons. Nobody likes an unnecessary trip to hospital but it is far better to raise a false alarm, especially with multiples, than to leave things too late. If you need any further incentive to act fast, remember that labour can progress very quickly, especially if your babies are small.

Dealing with premature labour

If you suspect premature labour, one thing you should do is avoid sex (and any strenuous activity), at least until you have checked with your doctor. Intercourse puts pressure on the cervix and the prostaglandins in semen may be enough to tip the balance and trigger full-blown labour.

Over the years, many measures have been devised to prevent or halt premature labour. They're not as reliable with twins and more, but they may buy a little time.

- Bed rest takes the weight off the cervix and helps improve placental blood flow, but on the whole hospital bed rest is of doubtful benefit.

- Cervical suture (tightening the cervix with a strong stitch) can help if the cervix is lax.
- Drugs like ritodrine, feneterol and terbutaline can be used, either by mouth or by injection. At various times, alcohol, nifedipine, magnesium sulphate and indomethacin (an anti-inflammatory drug) have also been prescribed despite lack of any obvious benefit in multiple pregnancy. New drugs are also being evaluated.

In fact, the proportion of babies born too soon has actually increased in the last two or three decades, but premature babies – multiples and singletons – are doing a lot better.

If you suspect your labour has started prematurely, ring the labour ward and go there right away. Once there, you might be assessed with a gentle internal examination, and you may have an ultrasound scan. Ultrasound estimation of the length of the cervix can be useful in assessing threatened pre-term labour: if the cervix has already shortened, labour is more likely to start. Your contractions and your babies' heartbeats will also be monitored for a while to see how things develop.

If you are in labour, you're likely to get one of the drugs mentioned. They're not for long-term use, but they may help for a while. Meanwhile you'll get an injection of steroid. This passes into the babies and within 48 hours helps their lungs to mature so that they'll be more ready for the outside world if they do arrive soon.

Another reason for going to hospital early with suspected premature labour is that it enables your babies to get swift specialised care during and after birth.

· *Labour* ·

Signs of labour include a show of mucus, when the plug is released from the neck of the womb as the cervix changes.

This can be the first symptom, and there may be some blood with it. If your waters break, you may lose clear fluid, either in a trickle or a gush. Get yourself to hospital if this happens, as there's a higher risk of cord prolapse with multiples. Or you might get regular contractions coming every 15 minutes or more often. Some women have low back pain or a dragging feeling in early labour.

If you are not sure you are in labour, it does no harm to check. Staff at the hospital can test any wetness to check whether it's amniotic fluid (as distinct from sweat or urine). On the labour ward, your contractions can be monitored, and your babies' heartbeats checked.

Whether your babies arrive on time or early, your labour is likely to be more high-tech than with singletons, so that complications can be spotted and treated promptly. Some women may find this medicalisation of childbirth off-putting, or even plain disappointing. Surely pregnancy and birth are natural, so why treat the process like the advanced stage of a dangerous disease?

Over the last 20 years or so, women have had greater choice in childbirth and have been able to reclaim the experience of becoming mothers. Women and their midwives have become more vocal and there has been something of a backlash against the traditional mechanistic – and often paternalistic – pattern of obstetric care. Midwives are once again the professionals with the lead role in normal pregnancy and labour. Meanwhile, doctors are increasingly questioning the part they themselves play and the results of their actions. The principles of what's called evidence-based medicine, or EBM, have influenced many different specialities all over the world, and obstetrics is no exception. However, when it comes to twins and higher multiples, there's less EBM to guide medical practice.

The trouble is that these pregnancies are less usual. You

have to accept that the human species is really only geared to producing one offspring at a time.

Good teamwork is the best approach for a woman in labour with twins. It may be that your twins will be delivered by a midwife, but with an obstetrician in attendance too, because labour is more traumatic for babies that are small or premature. There is also the higher risk of cord prolapse, for instance, and unusual positions. On very rare occasions twins can even lock: their presenting parts wedge together and make normal delivery impossible. For all these reasons, with twins and more you are about twice as likely to need help in labour, either with a caesarean or forceps.

That is not to say the birth won't be a joyous event, just that you should be prepared for it to be different from having one baby. The better prepared you and your partner are, the more likely the experience is to be satisfying. And if your doctor proposes any intervention in labour, you're entitled to know why.

Who will be at the birth?

If you have a named midwife, she may be there at the delivery, but this isn't always possible and there may be another midwife or even several of them during the course of your labour and delivery. Multiple births can pull a big crowd. Apart from the midwife and obstetrician, there will often be an anaesthetist for you and a paediatrician for each baby. There could also be many other nurses, midwives, junior doctors and possibly medical students, all determined not to miss the event.

Large numbers of people can be very off-putting, and some women may feel that an intimate moment has turned into some kind of show. Health professionals need to learn about multiple births, of course, but if you find the audience disturbing, tell your doctor or midwife as soon as possible.

You can decide about this, and other preferences you may have, in advance with your partner or birth companion, when you make a birth plan. Don't be too inflexible, though. In Tamba's survey of maternity services, 62 per cent of mothers made a plan in advance, but only a third were able to stick to it, and a further third stuck to it in part. Eighty-five per cent of the mums felt that the explanation they got for lack of choice was justified.

Method of delivery

Caesareans are far more common with twins. (The word comes from the Latin *caesus*, from the verb *caedere*, to cut, though commonly believed to refer to Julius Caesar – but his mother didn't have a caesarean!) In the UK, nearly 60 per cent of twins are delivered this way, compared with 25 per cent or so of singletons.

Triplets and higher multiples

Higher multiples are even likelier to be born by caesarean. The more babies you are carrying, the likelier it is that you will need intervention. Quads and more are almost always born by caesarean.

What is considered the best method varies with locality. In the USA, over 90 per cent of triplets arrive by caesarean. Within the UK there is a little variation from one hospital to another, but overall most triplets are born by caesarean. It may be reasonable to aim for a vaginal delivery if the first baby is head-down, but the trouble is that the way the second and third babies are lying can change during labour; they may therefore need help in a hurry. Furthermore, it's impossible to monitor three or more babies adequately in labour. Under the circumstances, there is logic in having a caesarean in the first place.

Presentation of twins

How your twins lie in the womb towards the end of your pregnancy is a major factor in deciding the most appropriate method of delivery. In about three-quarters of twin pregnancies, the first twin is head-down – what's known as a vertex or cephalic presentation.

About 40 per cent of twins are both head-down (vertex-vertex). Most of these could probably deliver normally, though their heart rates need close monitoring in labour for any signs of distress. In a recent national survey, 97 per cent of consultants in the UK would advise a vaginal delivery in this situation, unless the babies are premature. If you had a caesarean for a previous birth, there is still a chance that your twins can be born vaginally, just as long as your last caesarean was for a one-off reason, not for a permanent condition like a small pelvis.

In about 35 per cent of twins, the first is head-down but the second is breech (bottom-down), which is where things start getting complicated. The danger for a breech baby is that he cannot breathe as soon, because his head is born last. A breech baby is sometimes turned around in labour, either internally or externally, under ultrasound control. If your second twin is breech, you may still be able to have a vaginal delivery, unless:

- you had a previous caesarean, for whatever reason (it may not be safe to turn a breech around in a womb that has a caesarean scar)
- there are complications, like fetal distress.

The same survey showed that 68 per cent of obstetricians would advise vaginal delivery for a vertex-breech combination of twins.

In about 25 per cent of twins, the first baby is a breech. Here a caesarean is often done without the mother going into labour at all.

If you need a caesarean, both babies are born this way. It is unusual – though not unheard of – for the first twin to be born vaginally and the second by caesarean because a problem crops up in labour. You might groan at the thought, but midwife Debbie Sen's findings show that, surprisingly, many women to whom this happens don't find it a negative experience.

Forceps are used less than they once were, but they are a bit more common for twin births than for singletons, especially for the second twin. They help either to rotate a baby's head into a better position, or to get him out more quickly if distressed. A suction instrument called a ventouse can do some of the same work as forceps. However, it is not used for very small or premature babies because their heads are too vulnerable to withstand the suction pressure.

As you can see, exactly what happens depends not just on how the babies lie, but also on the length of the pregnancy before labour starts, and on factors which vary from woman to woman. An ultrasound may, for instance, have shown placenta praevia, a condition in which one or other placenta lies so low down in the womb that normal labour is impossibly dangerous. In this case, an elective caesarean is the only option.

Obstetric practice also varies a little from hospital to hospital, so you need to discuss with your specialist what is likely to happen in your case. Incidentally, the percentages given above are only approximate and they don't add up to 100 because not all babies are breech or vertex. Some are transverse, meaning that they lie horizontally across the uterus and therefore need a caesarean.

Pain relief

There are several methods, including:

- 'gas and air' (the gas is nitrous oxide; Entonox is nitrous oxide and oxygen)

- pethidine by injection (if given within two hours or so of delivery, this may affect the babies' breathing just after birth, especially the second twin's)
- pudendal block (local anaesthetic is injected deep into the pelvis; it is sometimes used for forceps or ventouse delivery, though an epidural is usually preferable)
- epidural injection (described below).

There are also drug-free methods, such as transcutaneous nerve stimulation (TNS or TENS). Relaxation should not be dismissed either – it is helpful in early labour.

Before they go into labour, some women decide that they want as little pain relief as possible, or even none. A few think that only a truly natural (often very painful) birth is a good birth, and anything less is a cop-out.

With twins and higher multiples, it's difficult for the process to be entirely natural anyway. Moreover, pain can be downright counter-productive. It can result in uncoordinated contractions which slow down labour and reduce placental blood flow to your babies. Pain also inhibits your own stomach from emptying, increasing the risk of your bringing up acid. This is potentially very dangerous for you.

Once pain no longer intrudes, you could also feel a lot calmer and able to enjoy labour, and that's got to be good.

Epidurals

In an epidural, local anaesthetic is injected into the spinal epidural space around the nerve fibres to numb them during labour. Hospitals differ in what they can provide, but many more of them now offer epidural facilities.

There's no doubt that the epidural has been the greatest advance in pain control in the last generation. It is the only method – barring general anaesthetic – that can totally abolish labour pains. Unlike a general anaesthetic, however, you are conscious and feel in control. Epidurals have special advantages for women with multiples:

- An epidural is ideal for a breech delivery.
- The second baby can change position after the first twin is born. Turning him without an epidural or general anaesthetic would be excruciating.
- With an epidural in place any other sort of intervention (e.g. forceps or a caesarean) that you may need can be done without a potentially dangerous delay.
- A caesarean under epidural rather than general anaesthetic allows you and your partner not to miss the first precious moments with your babies.

As a woman expecting twins, you may therefore be strongly advised to have an epidural during labour. In Tamba's survey, 58 per cent of women had an epidural. It may or may not be what you originally had in mind for your labour, but women who have had epidurals are usually very pleased with their effect.

The procedure

You will be lying on your side, with your knees and head bent. The anaesthetist injects a little local anaesthetic into the skin of your back, which stings momentarily.

Then he or she guides a very fine tube between two vertebrae (lumbar vertebrae number three and number four) in the middle of the back and into the epidural space, through which nerves travel outwards from the spinal cord to the rest of the body. These nerves carry sensation back to the spinal cord and up to the brain, where pain is ultimately 'felt'. To check that all is well, a test dose of anaesthetic is used at this stage.

Once in place, an epidural can be topped up with long-acting anaesthetic as needed, tailoring the dose to your requirements. For a caesarean, for instance, a fairly large dose is used, but for a vaginal delivery the anaesthetic can be allowed to wear off a bit so that you can feel the urge to push in time with your contractions. Epidurals can also help with pain relief after delivery.

The downside

You may have some worries about epidurals, but about 90 per cent of them are satisfactory overall. Research shows that back pain, which some women think of as a complication of labour, is not more common after epidural. However, nothing in medicine is without some disadvantage, and epidurals do have potential problems:

- Blood pressure tends to fall with an epidural. To counter-act this, you need a drip in your hand or arm, so you'll be a bit less mobile as a result.
- The most common difficulty is that the epidural may not work completely, though this is less likely with an experienced anaesthetist. Occasionally, numbness is patchy or only on one side of the body, which means that another method of pain relief has to be considered.
- While an epidural is being set up, there is a small risk of the needle piercing a membrane called the dura. This releases a few drops of cerebro-spinal fluid (CSF). It may sound frightening, but all it means in practice is that you may get a headache for a few days. Although it is not generally serious, the headache is pretty bad, and worse when sitting up. This obviously makes it harder to look after and enjoy your newborn babies, but it passes.

You may have heard of so-called mobile epidurals. These use a slightly different combination of drugs from the standard epidural, and leave a woman more mobile, so that she can walk around in labour if she wants. The trouble is that you are probably not going to be as mobile with a twin labour because of the monitors, so the mobile epidural is not really an option.

Vaginal delivery

Twin births usually follow three main stages when delivery is through the vagina.

The first stage of labour begins with the start of contractions, and ends with full dilatation of the cervix (you can further divide the first stage into a latent stage, when the cervix dilates slowly to 3 cm (1 inch), and an active phase, during which dilatation progresses more rapidly to its full extent of 10 cm (4 inches)). The second stage begins at full dilation and ends with the delivery of the babies. The third stage is delivery of the placenta (or placentas).

The first stage: dilatation of the cervix

During the first stage, the cervix effaces, or thins, as it dilates. Contractions build up in strength and frequency, drawing up the lower part of the uterus, so that the vagina and the uterus form one continuous birth canal. During the welcome lulls between each contraction, rest assured that no ground is lost: the muscles of the womb do not stretch out again to their original length.

A baby's heart rate is one measure of how he is coping with labour. To make sure your babies are not getting distressed, their heart rates will be monitored continuously throughout. At the same time, your contractions are also monitored, often by an intra-uterine catheter, which is more accurate than an external belt.

There is much debate about monitoring in singleton labours, and many obstetricians believe less routine monitoring would work just as well, and be less intrusive too. However, the issue is different with twins, who have a riskier time during birth. They really do need to be monitored continuously. Usually the first twin has a scalp electrode attached to his head (it can also be attached to the bottom of a breech baby), while the second twin is monitored externally via a sensor strapped to your abdomen. Thus both heart rates are monitored electronically. This is not possible with higher-order multiples, however.

With all this equipment in place, you won't be able to get about as much as you might have liked. Don't count on wanting to walk around much, however. By the time you get to term, you could be large and uncomfortable and you may welcome a lie-down.

How long does the first stage take? A first-time mother (known as a primigravida or primip) tends to have a slower labour, but it is impossible to be dogmatic here. In general labour with twins takes no longer than with a single baby. These days you are not left to languish in established labour; it tends to get speeded up medically if things are slow.

The second stage: birth of the babies themselves

For the first baby's head to emerge, you will need to push along with the contractions and with your midwife's or doctor's instructions. If you have an epidural which numbs most or all of the sensation, watching the monitor can help you synchronise your efforts with the contractions.

There can also be a phase between the first and second stages called transition, during which contractions become very intense. Sometimes you can get severe nausea or feverishness. It's important not to push during transition, so your obstetrician or midwife will guide you through this.

In most cases, once the head is born, the rest of the body follows swiftly, and the cord is clamped and labelled. If necessary, the second twin's membranes are then ruptured artificially at this point. His birth usually follows within

20 minutes or less, thanks to some more pushing on your part.

Until the early 1990s or so, the interval between first and second twin was rarely allowed to extend beyond 30 minutes for fear that the second baby might go dangerously short of oxygen. This can happen, but nowadays it is clear that a longer interval (up to two hours) can be safe, as long as the baby continues to be monitored closely throughout. Naturally, though, you will not want too long a wait! Even a short time between your twins can sometimes make a difference. In Germany, a woman had one twin four minutes before midnight on 31 December 1999 and the second twin one minute into the new millennium.

If there are no medical problems, you should be able to cuddle your first baby and put him to the breast for his first suckle as soon as he is born. As well as being rewarding for you both, this can stimulate contractions and help the birth of the second twin.

The third stage: delivery of the placentas

After the second twin is born and his cord is clamped, and again labelled, both placentas are delivered. They either deliver naturally, or by gentle pulling on the cords. Occasionally the first twin's placenta arrives before the second twin is born.

Bleeding can be heavy after the birth of twins and higher multiples because the uterus is more stretched and therefore less good at contracting back to size. When a post-partum haemorrhage occurs, it can be frightening, but there is treatment for it.

Caesarean section

Since over half of all twins in the UK are delivered by caesarean section, and you might not otherwise be told much about the procedure, it is worth focusing on what could happen.

A caesarean can be carried out as a planned procedure, without you going into labour at all. This is known as an elective caesarean, and you might be advised to have one, perhaps because of the way your twins are lying, or in the case of placenta praevia, for example. Caesareans can also be a good idea for twins that are growing less well than expected, because they are likely to find a natural birth more of an ordeal. A caesarean can also be done in an emergency, usually because one or other baby has become distressed during labour, but sometimes because of some other problem.

Either way, the technique is much the same. What is more, although many women imagine it might be reversed, the order in which your twins are born with a caesarean is the same as if they had been born vaginally.

Caesareans are normally done through a horizontal cut about 15 cm (6 inches) long, below or near the bikini line. You will be lying on your back, slightly tilted to one side to avoid putting weight on your major blood vessels. The obstetrician carrying out the procedure usually tilts you away from him or herself (the assistant is the one who gets wet feet from your amniotic fluid). You will need a catheter for a few hours to drain urine from your bladder, but most women don't find this uncomfortable.

The operation itself will not start till you are properly anaesthetised, either with a general anaesthetic or with an epidural which has taken full effect. If you have an epidural, your partner can normally remain with you throughout the caesarean, though he will be asked to stay near your head, where he can sit and talk to you without getting in the doctors' way.

With an epidural you don't usually feel a thing apart from a gentle rummaging sensation, or perhaps a little pulling, once the surgeon has got through the skin. Generally this is not unpleasant, but if you find it painful, say so. You won't usually see anything either, because a sterile drape is erected as a screen at about the level of your chest, but of course you hear and see your babies as soon as they emerge. As long as they don't need immediate medical help, you can have one or both put on to your chest to let them suckle or just to hold them close. In fact you can usually hold or touch them momentarily even if they need to go to the Special Care unit.

If you have a general anaesthetic, your partner is not normally allowed to stay with you, but you could ask the staff. He might want to be there, if only to take pictures or a video of the big occasion. Alternatively, he may be allowed in as soon as they are born, to see them and hold them before you wake up.

For technical reasons, or through shortage of experienced anaesthetists or midwives at times when a hospital is very busy, a few women who have an epidural still end up having a general anaesthetic for their caesarean. This is understandably a disappointment, especially if it has been promised that an epidural will take care of every eventuality.

After a caesarean, you'll soon be back on your feet, though you stay in hospital for around five days or so. And you are not exempt from postnatal exercises. Since your pelvic muscles have to work hard in the last few weeks of pregnancy, you still have to get them in shape after the birth.

The downside

These days some women – and their doctors – seem very enthusiastic about caesareans. Elective caesareans are now much more in vogue than they were, perhaps especially with career women and the middle classes (sometimes accused of being 'too posh to push'). There are currently more caesareans done than ever and many obstetricians find this trend worrying.

The modern caesarean is very safe, but it is still an operation and it has its drawbacks:

- you feel more tired after the birth
- you usually lose blood from the vagina for longer afterwards
- there is a higher chance of a DVT (deep-vein thrombosis or clot in a leg vein) or PE (pulmonary embolus or clot in the lung) than after a normal delivery, so to reduce the risk you may have heparin, an anticoagulant, by injection
- it is harder to look after babies, and to breast-feed them, when you are recovering from surgery yourself
- you often cannot drive for a few weeks afterwards.

> *The next day I felt really faint when I went to the loo. I was told I'd lost a litre of blood during the caesarean. All the other mothers on the ward were able to push the cots on wheels about, but I couldn't for about 48 hours and even then I had trouble managing two. Not all the nurses understood the difficulties of coping with two babies after a caesarean.*

You cannot expect to feel as well as you would if your abdomen hadn't been cut, and tiredness is perhaps the biggest disadvantage. This can really matter when you have to cope with multiples and need all the strength and energy you can summon. Therefore, a caesarean, like any operation, should clearly not be done without good reason. On the other hand, none of the minuses should deter one from having a caesarean when it is necessary.

Most mothers who have caesareans are happy with them. Those, like myself, who have their babies under epidural tend to be the most satisfied, often describing their experience in glowing terms and commenting on the supremely happy atmosphere during the birth.

> *I hadn't even wanted an epidural, let alone a caesarean, but it*

was excellent. After the birth I was crying but this was because I was so happy. My husband and two of the staff seemed overwhelmed, too. Yes, the day my sons were born by caesarean was the best day of my life. It was then, and it still is true now, ten years on.

If you have a general anaesthetic, you may feel groggy for a day or so and you will certainly miss the big event and those early moments. On the other hand, it is only a few hours in the lives of your children and you will have time with them when you feel more alert.

Twin births at home

This is a tough topic for a medic like myself. On the one hand, I want women to know that they have a choice, and they're entitled to exercise it. Your own home is undoubtedly more cosy and more relaxing than a delivery suite. Twins can be born at home – at one time they all were. A few of the more experienced midwives are happy to be involved in home births of twins.

On the other hand, given the risks, I firmly believe all twins and higher multiples should be born in hospital. Birth is traumatic for babies, especially if they are small or growth-retarded. This is the main reason why the risk of twins dying around birth and in the first week of life is roughly four times greater than for singletons.

The risk of malpresentation, cord prolapse or other complications is high, which can necessitate urgent delivery. That's why the need for a caesarean or forceps is greater. You can't get an epidural service or other anaesthetics at home. You might need attention after the birth: there's a higher chance of having a post-partum haemorrhage, and that sometimes requires resuscitation as well as blood transfusion. Perhaps an argument that's more compelling to women is that at home you can't get specialist paediatric care for your babies.

Yes, you have a choice. You know which I hope you'll choose.

Chapter Four
YOUR NEWBORN BABIES

I can honestly say that, tiny, slimy and bloody as they still were, my two babies were both the most beautiful things I'd ever set eyes on.

· *What Newborn Babies Look Like* ·

Before graduating to parenthood, most people imagine all babies look the same, but they don't. They may be small and wrinkled, or chubby and Churchillian; they could be hairy and will probably be covered with a greasy white layer of vernix to protect them from amniotic fluid.

Your babies may not be much alike. Size can be one obvious difference. The average birth weight of twins is 2.5 kg (5 lb 8 oz), with boys being a bit heavier than girls and non-identical (fraternal, dizygotic, or DZ) twins slightly heavier than identicals. There is, however, considerable variation. Size differences are often greatest between identical (monozygotic, or MZ) twins, a fact which even some professionals do not realise.

Newborn triplets each weigh on average 1.8 kg (4 lb), but a quarter of them weigh less than 1.5 kg (3 lb 5 oz). Quads tend to weigh in at 1.4 kg (3 lb) each or less, but again this varies a great deal.

Your babies may have different-shaped bodies. One may be short and podgy while the other is long and lean. Only one thing is certain: you will adore them from the start. Or will you?

· *Bonding* ·

Mothers (and their partners) are sometimes overwhelmed by a rush of love for their baby as soon as they see him. Bonding refers to what a parent feels for a young baby, an emotional tug which is a one-way process, at least at first. It probably begins in the womb with the kicks and the hormone surges inside a pregnant woman's body. Strong positive family feelings often surface at the first ultrasound scan or when hearing a baby's heartbeat courtesy of the midwife's Doppler machine. Falling in love with two or more babies at once, though, can be less straightforward.

> *Here I was with two heavenly bodies while all my friends had one baby. It felt downright promiscuous.*

According to one piece of research, 71 per cent of mothers of singletons experience immediate love for their babies, but only 50 per cent of mothers of twins do. Bonding with more than one can be really hard if you didn't know until the birth how many you were having, though luckily this is very unusual nowadays.

Soon you will discover that your twins' smiles, tempera-ments or voices differ, but for now you need something very obvious to distinguish your babies and help you feel close – and not just an ankle tag that you have to decipher from two inches away. You can tell your babies apart quickly by:

- the colour of their blankets
- a soft toy in the cot
- ribbons on the cot-handles
- dressing them differently, especially when they are in the same cot.

When they are awake, spend time on eye contact and soft

murmurings. These mini-conversations serve a purpose. Your twins may not understand what you say, but they know your voice already. Although you can't expect them to respond yet, they will soon. If they are healthy enough to be on the ward with you, it is a good idea to keep your babies by you at all times, so that you can get to know them more quickly. The other plus is of course the security of knowing where they are. However, if you want your babies to be in the nursery at night so that you can sleep, it doesn't mean you're lacking in maternal instincts. I believe new mums, weary as they are from the birth, benefit from having a choice. In Tamba's large maternity services survey, 78 per cent of the mums were given a choice of where their babies slept at night, and 68 per cent were offered staff help at night with the babies.

There may be a window of opportunity just after birth when bonding is most likely to take place, or at least a best time for it to happen. The received wisdom is that you must be physically close to your babies and breast-feed them. However, this is not strictly true. Mums feel just as much for bottle-fed or adopted babies. One can even experience passionate emotions for a baby who is stillborn. So if circumstances force you apart from your babies for the first few hours or even days after birth, don't beat yourself up about it. You can still develop the ties that bind.

Bonding with triplets, quads and more

If you're a mother of triplets or more, you can be excused for feeling immense pride, but along with it you may be uneasy. Just how is it possible to get to know and love so many babies? Can one hug these tiny scraps without crushing them? (A worry fathers in particular may have.) The situation tends to be more difficult if one or more of them has to be in the SCBU (Special Care Baby Unit).

Bonding will happen, but it may take time. Meanwhile, you can only do your best. If you have help, arrange things so that you rotate which baby you have to yourself, to give both you and him precious time together.

Favourites

Parents often worry about having a favourite, and they don't always feel they can talk about it. Rest assured this is usually a passing phase. No two people are truly identical and we shouldn't be too surprised at feeling slightly differently about each one of our babies.

This is especially true when there are noticeable differences. There is often some favouritism early on with boy-girl pairs, or towards the more attractive twin. Or when one baby is more placid and the other harder to comfort. Studies carried out with Tamba also found that birth-weight differences were significant: 84 per cent of mothers of twins who expressed a preference favoured the heavier baby. Before the birth, mothers often anticipate that they will feel more tender towards the smaller twin, but (as midwifery researcher Jane Spillman discovered) this is not what usually happens.

Although there is no instant 'cure' for favouritism, nature usually ensures that a parent's emotions wax and wane. The best thing you can do is spend a little unhurried time with each of your babies, especially the one you relate to less well. Get someone (friend, parent, partner, midwife, trainee nursery nurse – anyone you trust) to look after the other one while you attend solely to the baby for whom you feel less. Even at this early stage, you will find that being with one baby without having to think about the other gives you the chance to have a one-to-one, something multiples rarely get. You don't have to fall in love with the baby instantly – in fact, you probably won't. Just get to know him a little as an individual so that your feelings can develop when they are ready. (There is more about favouritism and older twins in Chapter 9.)

I called bonding a one-way process, but even new babies respond to people, especially those who seem to like them. One piece of research suggests that babies even share adult perceptions of attractiveness, preferring faces which are reasonably nice-looking. Perhaps it is worth smiling at your twins! One new mother said, 'I'd heard that babies liked happy faces better than grumpy ones, so I tried to make a big effort, even in the special care unit.'

Understandably, the death of a twin in pregnancy or soon after birth can be a huge obstacle to bonding with the survivor. Mixed feelings are normal at this time, a topic covered in detail in Chapter 15.

Fortunately, bereavement is something that very few parents go through. Far more often, one or more babies has to go to SCBU, the Special Care Baby Unit. However short their stay is, it makes it harder to feel close to your babies.

In the Special Care Baby Unit (SCBU)

In Tamba's survey, 40 per cent of twins and over 97 per cent of triplets spent some time in the neonatal unit or SCBU. Twins stayed an average of 14 days and triplets nearly twice that long. Your babies will usually need the specialised care of SCBU if they:

- weigh under 1.7 kg (about 3 lb 8 oz)
- were born before 32 weeks of pregnancy
- inhaled meconium (their immature bowel contents) during labour
- have fits
- are jaundiced
- have a major infection or some other specific problem.

Medical care

The concept of special care is simple: to duplicate the care the babies would have had in the womb. Premature babies need:

- warmth and moisture
- nourishment
- protection from infection.

Incubators come in several versions. Some have open tops and an overhead heater, while others are closed see-through boxes with full climate control and hand-sized port-holes for getting to the baby.

Premature babies are likely to have phototherapy: treatment with a blue light to break down the yellow pigment bilirubin. This combats the jaundice which is usual (but sometimes harmful) in babies born too soon.

A premature baby may need special feeding via a tube or even a vein. Some babies need more intensive care. Breathing difficulties are common because immature lungs lack a chemical called surfactant. Without it, a baby has to make a huge effort to get air into the lungs, which can lead to a condition called respiratory distress syndrome (RDS). For this reason, among others, a premature baby may need a ventilator to breathe for him.

Whatever treatment your babies have, they will be closely monitored. A blood gas monitor (oximeter) can be attached to a baby's hand or foot to monitor oxygen levels in the blood. Apnoea alarms are monitors that sound if a baby pauses too long between breaths. Using a combination of machinery and manpower, it is possible to keep a constant watch on a baby's blood pressure, heart rate, fluid balance and oxygen levels. Some parents are horrified to find that one or other baby is barely visible within an arsenal of machines and monitors, and are bewildered to hear alarms sounding so often.

Although the concept behind special care may not be complicated, the sophisticated technology used to deliver it can be daunting until you are familiar with it.

> *My boys spent 10 days in Special Care, the worst 10 days of my life. It was a complete roller coaster of emotions. I lived in fear of the worst while the staff constantly told me how well our boys were for 32-weekers. What says it all is that in every photo my face is hidden from view. I couldn't let anyone see my fear. They're five years old now – and doing grand.*

Will your babies be all right? It is a highly emotional time and this question is bound to prey on your mind. The only honest answer is that it depends on their individual situation. Please remember that there have been huge advances in what is called neonatal (newborn) medicine and nursing. For instance, doctors can now give chemical surfactant to help premature lungs develop. Ventilators can sense an infant's own weak efforts at breathing and synchronise with it. Recent developments in ultrasound and MRI mean that scans of a baby's skull can tell paediatricians what is going on inside it and help predict any risk of handicap. The downside is that there are many more tests and procedures to worry a parent. The huge upside is that you have excellent grounds for optimism.

The survival rate for small vulnerable babies is now much improved, and fewer than ever before will have any long-term disability. Twenty years ago, only a fifth of babies survived if they arrived weighing less than 1 kg (2 lb 2 oz, the same as the average jar of marmalade or bag of sugar). Now four-fifths or more survive. What's more, the outlook for premature twins is slightly better than for a prem singleton at the same stage. Twins have less respiratory distress syndrome, fewer congenital (inborn) abnormalities, and therefore a higher survival rate. You have triplets? Recent studies show that triplets too often fare much better than expected.

From 28 weeks onwards, the outlook for a baby is usually good But that doesn't mean babies born before then necessarily do badly. The premature baby charity BLISS funded research that shows that of all prem babies born before 25 weeks, half have no disability at all. And just look at the photos in the unit – almost every SCBU has a noticeboard covered with success stories in the form of pictures of healthy, smiling children, all previous patients who survived and are now enjoying life to the full.

What can a parent do in the special care unit?

If your babies are going to the SCBU, remind the staff that you want to touch them or hold them – even just for a moment – before they are taken to their incubators.

Although you may not be able to cuddle your babies much once they are in the SCBU, there is still a lot you can do for them:

- Most units will offer you a Polaroid of your babies, so even if you have no crib next to you on the postnatal ward, you will have a picture. Ask about taking your own photos or a video, if you can do this without using a flash or getting in the way.
- As soon as you can, start spending time in the unit. If you had a caesarean recently, someone can take you to Special Care in a wheelchair if necessary.
- Get to know which incubator is which at a glance. Make sure staff tell you if they move your babies around the unit.
- You may want to breast-feed your babies, and this is often possible (by expressing milk) even when they are in Special Care. The next chapter has a section on breast-feeding babies in SCBU. Some premature babies benefit from a special supplement of vitamins, minerals and protein added to breast milk to help their growth.
- If your babies are having bottles, you could help too. Talk

to the nursing and medical staff as soon as you can about feeding. When a baby has already been started on bottles, it is possible, but more difficult, to breast-feed him later.

- Your babies need to feel and smell you, and vice versa. So touch your babies, if necessary through the incubator port-holes. It will feel unnatural to begin with, but frequent touch is good for you and your babies. A still hold can be better than stroking or patting. You can also hold hands. This way you will gradually get to know each other. Even very young babies can recognise a mother's touch. You will also gain confidence in handling them, which helps bonding. Once your babies are sturdy enough, skin-to-skin care has a very positive effect, and can help a baby's breathing and general health. You may be able to hold both babies to your chest together, or you may need to do this separately with each. Whichever you do, be careful with any tubes or cables attached to them, and get a nurse to help with positioning. There's more about the benefits of skin-to-skin (also called kangaroo) care in Chapter 5 in the section on breast-feeding.

- If only one of your babies is unwell, you can feel torn between the one in Special Care and the one on the ward – and they may be a long trek apart. Maybe you are concerned about the welfare or safety of the one left unattended while you visit the special care unit. It is vital for mothers to have their twins close together, so ask. Perhaps you and the healthier baby can at least be moved to a ward nearer the SCBU.

- Ask if you can take the well baby with you to visit his twin. This may not mean much to him, but it often makes mothers feel better. Older siblings can often visit too, though bear in mind they can quickly get tired or bored by the whole thing.

- If possible, get photos or videos of the babies together to reinforce their twinship. This, says midwife Jane Spillman, is terribly important to mothers, especially when one baby is ill.

- Small-for-dates or prem babies may be less attractive even to their own parents (mums often feel this though they may not like to admit it). Try not to mind about the odd flake of dried blood or bits of vernix. It's better to leave these be than to wash or pick them off.

- When only one baby is unwell, nurses may encourage you to concentrate on the healthy baby, but your sicker twin needs your care and attention – and so do you. Rest assured that your well twin won't suffer as a result. If you want to be alone with the sicker one, say so. On the other hand, some mothers like the companionship of a friendly, capable nurse when they handle a very sickly baby.

- You may be afraid of developing feelings in case your baby dies, leaving you more distressed than if you had never become attached to him, but this is not borne out by the experience of parents who have been bereaved. In fact, they cherish whatever contact they had before they lost their child. If you have this type of worry, talk to staff on the unit. Paediatricians are usually experienced in these matters, and there are also counsellors attached to special care units.

- Ask about your babies' treatment and get involved in their care. There may be lots of day-to-day tasks you can take on, especially as your babies get stronger. Hospital policy has changed a lot – and so has the thinking on infection. Changing a tiny baby's nappy for the first time can be scary, but you'll soon get the hang of it, and will value the contact with your baby.

- On the unit, you will get to know other parents over snatched cups of tea, but don't assume that what is happening to their babies applies to yours. Always ask the doctors or nurses for information about your situation. You could keep a notebook of your babies' progress and jot down important points – use different pages or sections for each of your babies. You can also get general information and support from BLISS (see Resources, page 373).

- Make sure your partner doesn't get left out. Fathers are often shocked when their baby is in SCBU, but people rarely ask how he is coping.

Will my babies grow?

If your babies are small, you may wonder whether they will ever catch up. This is a tough question to answer, but it needs to be addressed because so many mothers of small or prem babies want to know, and yet are afraid to ask because they anticipate a disheartening reply.

Size does matter to mums and dads. It is vital to parents of multiples when only one baby is small because the difference between a tiny mite of an infant and his bouncing sibling of the same age is very obvious to all concerned.

It's usual to monitor the long-term growth of any child born small or premature. As a rule, small babies grow well if they are small only because they were born too soon. The more premature they are, the longer they take to catch up, so if your babies are both (or all) small because they arrived two months prematurely, you can expect the early disparity to vanish over the next couple of years. Twins tend to catch up in weight very rapidly, especially in the first few months, when they can gain faster than singletons.

There are a few exceptions, for instance when the placenta functions less well, or if there was twin-to-twin transfusion syndrome (see Appendix, page 348). If a baby happens to be unduly small for the length of time spent in the womb, he may not do much catching up. A baby very much smaller than her twin (or her co-triplets) could remain petite. This is especially true when a baby faces a lot of medical problems as a newborn.

Babies do confound the issue by coming in various shapes and sizes, but you can get a rough idea of a baby's growth potential from his length. If he is underweight for the age at which he was born but is a good length, he may make up his weight easily, often within a few weeks of birth.

When can I get them home?

It is hard to say exactly, apart from the obvious answer 'When they are ready'. Whenever they come home, however, this is the next phase of the biggest adventure of your life.

The smaller or more premature your babies are, the likelier it is that you will have to leave one behind in hospital when you go home. Many units do their best to keep both babies together instead of creating chaos for you by discharging them at different times, but unfortunately hospital services are often fully stretched.

Occasionally babies are even in different hospitals. This is far from ideal from a parent's point of view, obviously, and you are entitled to make a noise about it. Again, though, it can't always be helped, especially with triplets or more. Despite the practical problems, try to visit as much as possible. The more distant baby is still part of the family and needs to take his place in it as soon as he can. Talk about your baby to any friends or relatives who cannot visit him. You may have difficulty bonding with the sickest baby, so don't expect to feel instant love for him.

On the other hand, some mothers find that having one baby home at a time gives them a welcome chance to get adjusted to each one separately.

Yes, it was very hard having each of my triplets discharged from hospital at different times, but I don't know how I would have managed had they all come home together, needing three-hourly feeds.

Chapter Five

FEEDING AND OTHER IMMEDIATE PRACTICALITIES

Plan for twins or triplets like an army campaign. Before the babies come home, stock the freezer, buy ten times as much detergent and fabric conditioner as you think you might need, and have leaflets for your local takeaway. Get on the internet and have nappies, formula and groceries delivered to you by your local supermarket.

· Feeding Your Babies ·

When they have their first scan, many women give up the idea of breast-feeding because they think they can't nourish two or more babies. Of course it is perfectly feasible and mothers have successfully breast-fed twins for centuries – there was no other way. Today, I wish more of my fellow professionals would realise that it is possible, and desirable, to breast-feed multiples.

For those who were built compactly, the size of your breasts does not determine your success in breast-feeding. One new mother recalls how hurt she felt when told by the midwife, inaccurately as it turned out, that she would never have enough milk.

Breast-feeding twins is, however, more demanding than with a singleton. Be honest with yourself and, however you decide to feed your babies, don't feel guilty or pressurised.

Naturally, this is easier said than done, especially if it is your first pregnancy, but you need to be at ease with your decision.

Although it's now usual to put a baby to the breast immediately after birth to get breast-feeding established, it is not essential, so don't be despondent if you miss the chance to do this. And don't rely too much on previous experience of breast-feeding. Milk can flow more freely the second time around.

Baby formulas have improved beyond recognition in recent years, and of course it is perfectly possible to grow healthy babies with them. However, as a living thing, breast milk is still superior. It has special benefits for twins, triplets or more, so I encourage you to give it a go.

In favour of breast-feeding

- The perfect food for babies in terms of nutrients, breast milk also contains antibodies which protect against infection. And colostrum contains immune cells which will colonise a baby's gut and protect against both infection and allergy. Breast-feeding is especially good in the first three or four months, before a baby produces his own antibodies.
- Premature babies benefit especially, because they can have trouble digesting.
- Breast milk protects against severe gastro-enteritis, partly because of the antibodies it contains and partly because it requires no fiddly preparing.
- Because of the essential fatty acids in it, breast milk is best for brain development, especially in premature babies. Research suggests intelligence is a few points higher than in bottle-fed infants.
- Breast-fed babies are thought to suffer less eczema and/or asthma, but this is not proven.
- Breast-feeding seems to protect against cot death (SIDS or sudden infant death syndrome).

- Breast-fed babies need less 'winding'.
- Breast-feeding brings you physically (and possibly emotionally) closer to your babies. As a result your babies may be more satisfied, though like everything in parenting there are no guarantees.
- Because it is a supply-and-demand arrangement, you are unlikely to overfeed.
- Breast-feeding helps the womb contract back to its normal size. Because it burns calories, you could regain your figure more easily, but be prepared to be patient on this one. The jury is still out as to whether it protects against breast cancer in later life.
- It is cheaper than bottle-feeding, though you have to eat and drink more.
- Breast-feeding needs negligible advance preparation for each feed, and outings are that much easier.
- Full breast-feeding (i.e. without any formula) gives some protection against pregnancy, but don't bank on it, especially since mothers of multiples are more fertile.
- Last but not least, breast-feeding feels lovely. It can be an intensely sexual experience.

In favour of bottle-feeding

- Someone else can easily feed your babies. This gives others (your partner, for example) a chance to be involved in their care and it gives you an opportunity to do something novel, like shop, go back to work or look after your other children. Or sleep.
- You don't get sore nipples.
- You can still cuddle your babies and hold them close.
- You know how much nourishment they are getting. On average, every 24 hours a baby needs 2–3 fl oz of formula milk for each pound he weighs (100–170 ml per kg). Babies vary, so this is just a rough guide.

- Since you don't have to bare your breasts several times a day and you don't leak (after the first few days), you can wear what you want.
- You can feed your babies wherever you like (in winter, breast-feeding can be inconvenient, if not downright cold).
- Bottle-feeding demands special equipment and preparation (and greater cost) but is less taxing physically. It's possible that you will return to your normal mental state more quickly; you will sweat less at night, too.
- Your babies may sleep through the night more soundly. A breast-fed baby could be waking at night not just for a feed, but for a 'human dummy' as well, which may perpetuate the habit.
- Older siblings may be less jealous.

All in all, it is a personal decision which depends on you and your lifestyle. If you are still unsure, try talking to an expert from La Leche League or the NCT, or Tamba Twinline can put you in touch with another mum who has successfully breast-fed. A mother of twins can breast-feed if she sets her mind to it. You may have been put off if you had a caesarean, but the method of delivery doesn't really impact on your chances of successful breast-feeding. Other things being equal, you could start by breast-feeding. Even some breast milk is better than none. You can always change to bottles later, but once babies start sucking from an artificial teat it can be very hard to win them over to the breast.

If your babies are separated from you because they go to SCBU or perhaps just the night nursery, they may be given something other than your breast milk. Nowadays this happens less often, but, just to be sure, make staff aware of your wishes. It is possible to give breast milk to even very small or prem babies, and this is covered later in this chapter. If you plan to breast-feed but you can't yet for whatever reason, and your babies need artificial feeds, ask if they can be fed from a cup.

Even premature babies as young as 30 weeks or so can often manage cup feeds as long as the right technique is used. This helps avoid so-called nipple confusion, when a baby who has been started on bottles has trouble switching to the breast.

· *Breast-feeding Twins* ·

A friend boasted that she could have read War and Peace *while breast-feeding her baby. But I couldn't read anything while feeding my twins because I didn't have a hand free to turn the pages. I watched a lot of TV though.*

The principles of nipple care and latching on are the same with twins as with a single baby, and your midwife, antenatal clinic or breast-feeding counsellor can give you general information, so go to any teaching sessions on offer. This section concentrates on areas that are of special interest to the mothers of twins.

A routine is vital when you have more than one baby, and you need to get into one as early as possible. All the same, it is usual to begin by feeding new babies on demand: whenever they seem hungry. This is important because you build up a supply of milk based on how much the babies suckle. If your twins are very small or premature, you may be advised to feed them every two or three hours, regardless of whether or not they are hungry.

To save time, it is normal to feed both babies simultaneously unless there is a good reason not to. If one wakes for a feed, rouse the other one. He may not take much at this feed, but with luck the babies will eventually synchronise. The other advantage of feeding both at the same time is that the other breast will not leak uselessly, as it often does when feeding a singleton. You may want to feed your babies separately if they are of very different sizes and hence have different food needs.

However, separate feeds are useful in the early days of feeding, when you are getting used to it all, and they bring the bonus of giving you special time with each baby individually. Some mums continue feeding their twins separately despite time constraints. A few use their free hand to read a book or hug their singleton toddler (second twin permitting). There is no law that dictates you should feed them simultaneously, and you will find what works for you.

Apart from this, the most obvious difference when breast-feeding twins is positioning. Some mothers have them in the same position as a single baby (as shown in the diagram), but this gives no control over their bodies; they may also kick each other throughout the feed.

The more popular position for twins is the 'rugby football' hold shown. This allows you to control their bodies a bit, you are cuddling them more and their legs don't get in the way.

Some mothers compromise and have their babies more or less parallel during feeds, which can work well. As you will find for yourself, there are other possibilities too.

Your own comfort is crucially important. You are likely to be feeding for several hours a day, which puts immense strain on your neck, shoulders and back. Your back needs to be supported and your babies raised to nipple level. Many mothers find a large V-shaped or triangular cushion essential, but other cushions or pillows will work as long as the whole arrangement is secure. Wherever you do this, have a big glass of water or juice within reach. Breast-feeding is thirsty work. As for the phone, it's probably best to use an answering machine to start with, though in time you may be able to free up a hand to deal with calls.

A good place to feed twins is on a sofa or bed. Single beds are usually too narrow to accommodate you, babies and cushions without something vital falling off; this is a common difficulty in hospital. Despite this, do try feeding both babies

Some positions for breast-feeding twins

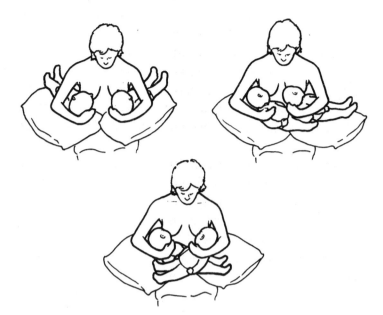

together before you leave hospital, as you will have more help on hand than at home. On a single bed, you may be better off sitting sideways on, but make sure your back is supported. What seems comfortable to begin with can change over the next twenty minutes or half-hour, especially if one or other baby comes off the nipple and has to be helped to latch on again.

Getting and keeping the babies securely latched on is the main difficulty to begin with, and you may feel you don't have enough arms. As a novice, it is difficult to juggle two wet sponges. While you are still in hospital, get a midwife to stay with you throughout the feed, to give you a hand in case one baby comes off the nipple in mid-feed. One baby may have more trouble latching on. If so, get this one positioned on the breast first. Then your helper can hand you his twin to put on to the other breast.

Premature babies tend to suck less well, especially if born before 34 weeks or so. Small babies can also be hard to feed if you have big breasts which seem to engulf them. The opposite is not easy either: if you have smallish breasts and fairly big babies it can be awkward to get comfortable, particularly if the babies take it into their heads to wriggle during the feed.

Once you've got the hang of it, though, you will do fine on your own. You can have one baby at the ready on the sofa next to you while you put the other one on to the breast. That way you can more easily scoop up the waiting baby for his feed, without letting go of the one who is already latched on.

You may hit a snag with maternity and nursing clothes. Of what use is just one limited opening down the middle? It is sometimes possible to find night-dresses with two slits, one over each breast. Or you could just choose tops you can unbutton completely or lift up. Some mothers do not like exposing themselves to this extent, but others couldn't care less.

Some mums swap breasts at each feed, while others keep one breast for each baby. Since babies don't always need the same amount, you can get lopsided, albeit temporarily. If your babies are very different in weight, you may prefer to alternate breasts. A safety-pin on your bra strap can remind you which breast to give a particular baby at the next feed – the smaller one, say, can be the safety-pin baby.

For how long should you feed at each session? The usual answer is however long the babies want. However, they may want to go on sucking for comfort long after they have got all the feed they need, and you could end up with sore nipples, which will put you off the whole thing. In general, fair-skinned women can stand less sucking. It is best to feed as often as the babies seem to want, but if you cannot manage to let them suck for as long as they want, rest assured that five to 10 minutes at the breast per feed will usually drain most of the milk.

You can always express milk if your breasts are engorged, or you want someone else to feed for you, perhaps if your babies are in the Special Care unit. Even if they are not in SCBU, it is useful to know how to express, and you should be shown how to do this before you leave hospital. The principles are exactly the same as for singleton mums. If you express milk more than just occasionally, a hand-operated breast pump may not be enough and could be laboriously slow. You can hire an electrical one from the NCT, or ask the hospital. Most women who have tried one say the machine makes them feel like a cow, but they often add, 'So what?'

In the weeks and months that you are breast-feeding, make sure you have plenty to drink. Guinness is the stuff traditionally recommended, although it is probably no better or worse than other high-calorie fluids. A drop or two of alcohol may help to relax you but too much could be harmful to your babies. Make sure you eat enough, too, especially protein and carbohydrate. Nature has a way of fixing things, and the best plan is just to eat when you are hungry. Now is not the time to diet.

As a guide, you will need 800–1,000 calories a day more than a non-breast-feeding mum (that's 400–500 calories for each baby). You needn't drink a lot of milk yourself, though milk and dairy products do have the benefit of containing lots of protein and calcium. Make sure you have plenty of the main food groups, just as you did in pregnancy. The major difference is that now you don't need to avoid liver, pâté, soft ripened cheeses and cook-chill meals. If there are many allergies in your family, steer clear of peanuts and other nuts while breast-feeding. Three main meals and three snacks a day should do the trick, and don't skimp on this even though you're short of time.

You may want to breast-feed for just a few weeks, or for

months on end. Whatever you can manage will benefit the babies. Many mothers have successfully fed their twins on breast milk till the end of the first year. If you are happy with it, and the babies are thriving, there is no reason why you shouldn't too. Alternatively, you may want to stop when they start solids at four to five months. This is often a time when their requirements increase anyway, so it's harder to keep up with breast-feeds. This stage can also be messy, as babies usually smear solids on to themselves, and then on to you and your clothes.

There may be other times when you want to top up with a bottle of formula milk, which is known as complementary feeding. A bottle of either formula or expressed breast milk is ideal for giving you a little time away from your twins. The snag with bottles of formula – apart from having to prepare them – is that a baby then sucks less from the breast, decreasing the milk supply. If you are going to offer formula as well, make sure you do so just after a breast-feed, not before.

As a long-term arrangement, mixing breast and bottle works well for some. Admittedly you have the drawback of making up bottles and still need the commitment for breast-feeding. On the other hand, the babies still get the well-known benefits of your own milk and the special closeness of breast-feeding. Mixing breast and bottle can enable a mother to breast-feed when she would otherwise have given up.

If you have a partner, his support is vital to breast-feeding twins successfully. At first you may simply need help in getting set up and moral support if things aren't going smoothly, but even later on, when you are skilled at it, breast-feeding multiples is still a commitment. It is time-consuming for your partner, not least because you will need to rest more than if you only had one baby. Meanwhile, the number of chores to do is at least double that for a singleton. Any extra hands on board with household matters will help boost your milk output. Rest is vital to lactation. If you find your production flagging, it's not because you're fated to fail but because you're trying to be superwoman.

Unfortunately even today some midwives and other professionals can be negative, or offer only token support if you're breast-feeding twins. In Tamba's maternity survey, about a quarter of mums didn't get the help and understanding they needed with breast-feeding. Despite this, 73 per cent managed to breast-feed or express milk for a week – even among the caesarean group, 71 per cent did.

You can get more advice on breast-feeding from the NCT breast-feeding helpline and La Leche's 24-hour advice line. A visit to another mother who is breast-feeding twins can be very helpful. There will be times when breast-feeding is easy and other times when it is something of a struggle. It can take weeks to establish, but if you are determined to succeed, then you almost certainly will. Take encouragement with every passing day. Each is a small landmark, and you can congratulate yourself on that.

· *Breast-feeding Triplets* ·

I can't begin to describe the sense of achievement I got from breast-feeding my babies for three whole months.

There are no biological reasons why a woman's milk can't stretch for three infants, only practical hurdles. One very obvious obstacle: a woman has a maximum of two nipples. Breast-feeding your triplets is still a very good idea. You will be very short of time, obviously, but breast-feeding gives you a chance to cuddle up to your babies, and, being generally smaller and more premature than twins, triplets (and more) can benefit even more dramatically from the goodness of breast milk. The down side is:

- your babies are more likely to be in the SCBU
- they may not suck well if they are very premature.

Breast-feeding three is thoroughly exhausting, but many women have successfully managed it – and enjoyed it – for as long as six months or more. Tamba found that half their triplet mums breast-fed at least one of the babies. Their Supertwins Group can put you in touch with mothers who are happy to share their experiences and pass on practical advice. If you actually watch a mum breast-feed, it will convince you more eloquently than any book can. This is especially useful if you've come into contact with midwives or other professionals who think it cannot be done.

Your choice lies between:

- breast-feeding only one or two of the babies (perhaps the smallest or most vulnerable) and giving formula to the rest
- breast-feeding one or two babies and bottle-feeding the other(s), perhaps on a rota basis, so that every 24 hours all get breast-feeds and all get bottles
- breast-feeding two and giving your expressed milk to the third
- breast-feeding all three at different times (very time-consuming but entirely possible if you have help in the home).

If you have any sort of rota system for the feeds, you need to keep written notes. Otherwise you'll get hopelessly muddled, especially when you're half asleep.

You can use the positions and principles described above for breast-feeding twins. If you have a helper, he or she can take the third baby. Or you may be able to position him safely near you, even perched atop your V-shaped pillow. It can't escape your attention if he then starts to slide off.

To make a go of breast-feeding triplets, you really have to

put your own health first. Rest, healthy food and plenty to drink have to be your priorities. If you are not sure you are succeeding in nourishing three, weigh your babies more often, say twice a week. With triplets, your health visitor should be happy to come to your home to weigh the babies. If she doesn't offer, ask. Better still, insist.

Breast-feeding in the Special Care Unit

Even when your babies are premature, it's possible to breast-feed. If you don't want to breast-feed as a long-term solution, giving your Special Care babies breast milk can help them so much. Babies under 34 weeks of pregnancy can't suck well, so at first, your babies may get nutrients from a drip into the stomach (some very immature babies initially need feeding through a vein). If you express at this early stage, the colostrum you produce before the milk comes in is very valuable for their immunity.

Skin-to-skin contact is a great way to help each of your babies feel warm and loved in turn. Skin-to-skin, also called kangaroo care, means holding each baby gently against the bare skin of your chest and letting him snuggle. Babies often cry less and grow better if you spend time like this with them every day. It may also boost the quantity of milk you produce, and even its quality, because your immune system will respond to germs in your babies' environment. Nature can be amazingly kind when you least expect it.

A breast pump doesn't make more milk, at least not till the next session. It simply drains what's there, so the let-down reflex (described in all standard baby-care manuals) is still essential. That's why expressing or pumping often works better if you do it next to your babies' cots or incubators. If you need to express often, get into a routine as soon as possible. It's best done often and at regular intervals. Mums who express for all feeds can expect their total daily time with an electric pump to be around two hours, but this varies.

When you first give one of your babies a real breast-feed, just hold him close and do not make him feed. He will enjoy the contact and lap up your smells before he enjoys your milk. Once he is happy being there, he will start feeding. It sometimes helps to express a few drops of milk so that some of it is sitting on the nipple waiting for him. Or you can express directly into his mouth while someone holds him.

· *Bottle-feeding Twins or More* ·

Although bottles may seem the easy option, it is hard to get close to two or more babies and keep the bottles in the right position, let alone rub your nose if it happens to get itchy during a feed (surprising how often that happens). Again, the general principles are the same as for bottle-feeding any baby. With the current emphasis on breast-feeding, it is hard to get information on different formulas or instructions on preparing bottles, but your midwife can help if you ask. Mums who opt to bottle-feed should be shown in hospital how to prepare feeds. There are a few obvious differences when you have two or more babies.

Position

Finding the right position depends to a great extent on how big your babies are. Using cushions to support your arms, you will probably find it best to hold a bottle in each hand and have a baby on either side of you, either:

● alongside each of your legs
● with a head resting on each of your thighs
● or with a baby on each arm (you'll need supple wrists).

You could also prop the babies up side by side and hold their bottles rather than them, but then you won't be physically close to them, which is a distinct disadvantage.

With practice, you will soon settle on one position – or several – which you find most convenient. If there is another adult about, you can each feed a baby like a singleton. However short of arms you are, never leave a baby propped up with a bottle unsupervised.

Some positions for bottle-feeding twins

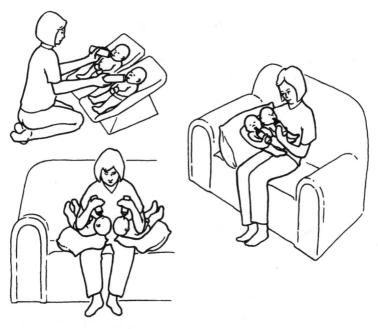

Timing

As with breast-feeding, your aim is to get into a regular routine as soon as you can, but you generally need to start off by feeding on demand. It is often best to feed twins simultaneously, waking the one who is not hungry yet. The one you've woken will probably look bewildered when you show him a bottle and may not take as much at this feed as the one who's howling for his, but it all works out after a while. However, if they are of very different weights, you risk overfeeding one of them, and you may be better off catering to their individual needs: feeding them separately from the start even though it takes longer. If this seems very time-consuming, tell yourself they're getting more than food – they're also having some precious one-to-one with you.

Preparing feeds

Preparing feeds up to 24 hours in advance is fine if you have enough bottles – and space in the fridge. As an alternative to storing individual bottles, you could use large measuring jugs full of formula. This needs to be stirred before pouring from it; use a sterile spoon.

Don't forget to shake bottles well before you give them, or you will end up with a thick sludge in the bottom of each bottle and water in each baby. You may be able to get by with one sterilising unit at first, especially if you have half-size bottles, but don't invest specially in these – they are not useful for long unless your babies are very tiny.

Two sterilising units (borrow one or more if you can) are better than using one huge container as they will be easier to lift and empty. Different-coloured bottles (for example, blue and red caps) are handy so you can remember which baby had what, particularly if you have to break off mid-feed. If any bottles are left more than an hour, assume they contain germs, and throw them out. Never reheat bottles.

Warming cold bottles

Many babies will accept cold bottles, but don't give cold feeds to very young or small babies. It will cool them down too much. Heat it up first. However, milk that is too hot is very dangerous. It can cause the lining of the back of the throat to swell up, which can asphyxiate and even kill a baby. A microwave oven may seem a good method for reheating bottles, especially when preparing two or more at a time, but this method can create hot spots in the milk, which can scald your babies. Instead use a bottle warmer or two, or just a bowl of hot water.

Another tip is to deliberately make up formula with insufficient water and add hot later when you want it. For instance, if your babies need 180 mls (6 fl oz), make bottles up in advance with enough scoops of powder for this amount, but only 120 mls (4 fl oz) of water, and leave them in the fridge. Just before you give the feed, add the remaining quantity of freshly boiled (hot) water. A little practice will enable you to get the proportions right. Of course, never give (or let anyone else give) formula that is too concentrated. If someone else will be feeding, the bottles should be carefully labelled to show that top-up is needed.

Whatever means you use for preparing feeds, test the temperature every time. The traditional way is to sprinkle a few drops on to the inside of your wrist.

· *Basic Equipment for Newborns* ·

By this stage you should already have the basics, like something for your twins to wear, but if you're deeply super-stitious or just got caught on the hop by delivering early, then you need to get some things. So send your bewildered partner out now for an emergency foray to the shops.

Those of you who already had one baby have some idea of what equipment is available – and what is actually needed, which is not at all the same thing. You can quickly fill up a house with so-called 'essentials' that hardly ever get used. With multiples, you obviously need some different items of equipment and may have less disposable cash.

Clothing

You need at least:

- vests: two or three for each baby
- stretch suits: at least three each (get ones that open down the front. The other kind is too fiddly)
- jackets: two each
- bonnets: one each (for winter, or if the babies are very small).

This really is the bare minimum. The more you have of these things, the easier life will be. Make sure everything is machine-washable and doesn't need ironing. Ideally, it should all go in the tumble-dryer. There are limits as to how much you can drape over the radiators.

If you have spare cash, get more of the basics, and forget about the fiddly finishing touches. Since time is precious, I wouldn't bother with bootees or mittens, no matter how adorable they look. Pram shoes are a complete waste of time, and often too rigid for tiny soft feet. Besides, twins can hurt each other by kicking with pram shoes on. Real outdoor shoes are superfluous until your babies begin to walk properly outside. Until then, all they need is padded slip-on elasticated footwear with non-slip soles. Later on, when buying the first pairs of proper shoes, have them measured expertly and choose, if you possibly can, an easy style with a Velcro closure, not buckles or laces.

At this early stage, other useful items are shawls (one each) and several 'dribble cloths' each (you can use terry nappies or muslin squares). These also come into their own to protect sheets and blankets.

Equipment

- baby bath (preferably with stand)

- nappy-changing bag or mat (preferably both)
- nappy-changing stand (to save your back, but you could use a changing mat on a chest of drawers)
- baby listener (can be very useful).

Cot

You can often manage with just one for six weeks or more, depending on the size of your twins. They can sleep side by side (see page 154). The advantage here is that the babies can both be positioned near the foot of the cot and the bed-clothes arranged to come up no higher than their shoulders (this is thought to be an important factor in preventing cot death). To save confusion at night, it helps to keep each baby in the same place, e.g. Daniel on the right and Sam on the left.

Car seats

One for each baby, if you have a car. You need seats for the trip home from hospital. Rear-facing baby seats are ideal for the very young and are usually suitable for babies weighing up to 13 kg (28 lb 8 oz). They generally have a handle so they can be removed and carried like a basket, even with a sleeping baby. The downside is that it's awkward to lug two of them. In the house, the car seat can double as reclining chair and may save you buying bouncing cradles (you would otherwise need one of these for each baby). Don't put a baby seat in the front of the car if you have a passenger airbag: in an emergency it can inflate so forcefully that it breaks a baby's neck.

You may prefer to hire rear-facing seats initially, then install traditional forward-facing child seats which are suitable from 9 kg (20 lb) upwards and will last throughout toddlerhood.

Baby slings

Useful if you and your partner intend to carry a baby each, but potentially damaging to your back if you are planning to carry two babies at a time yourself. It may be the only way you can get on a bus unaided, but your twins will soon get heavy, and what seemed like a manageable weight when you leave home can become unbearable 15 minutes later.

Pushchairs and buggies

For a short while you can often manage with a single pram, if you already have one, but soon your babies will be too big. A large second-hand twin pram can last you most of the first year and well into the second, but has the drawback that it may not fit into the car. Whether you need one at all depends on your lifestyle. Many double buggies and push-chairs are suitable for the very young – but they give less protection than a pram against the elements. The buggy may not be up to the job as your babies get bigger and heavier. If it gives up the ghost after a year or so, you will need to replace it. Then you can choose one that's more suitable for toddlers. Have a look too at Tamba's *Buggy and Pushchair Guide* (see page 376).

Side-by-side buggies are usually better than tandem models because twins can then see each other. Get a good, solid buggy that conforms to British Standards and one that is preferably new. It may have to work much harder than a buggy used for siblings of different ages. Before you buy, check the width (the crucial comparison is with the width of your front door or porch), weight, folding qualities and handle height of the models you are interested in. All-terrain sports buggies tend to be longer than average. Try getting one with a rain-hood that can stay on even when you fold the buggy. If you are not sure exactly what you want, you could hire one first. Incidentally, you still need a buggy even if you drive everywhere. If you carry both babies to the car, how will you open the car door? It is much safer to put them both in their buggy for the 30 metres or whatever to the car than take them out of the house one by one. If you have a toddler already, you can get a buggy board that fits on to the double buggy for him to stand on and get a ride. It makes the buggy a lot heavier, though.

Triple buggies can also be side-by-side (here, width gets even greater and you have to consider shop entrances) or have one seat in front. You could make do, for a while anyway, with a double buggy and a sling for one baby.

Car

No, I am not suggesting you have to splash out on a new car now, but when you do have a choice, you'll find a four-door model much easier. With a really big litter to carry, this may be the moment you are forced to give up dreams of the sporty low-slung number and consider something like a minibus or people-carrier (MPV).

Buying second-hand can work out well with equipment for twins and more, and local twins' clubs often have used things on offer. If you buy things in this way, or borrow equipment from friends, make sure everything's safe and in good clean condition. In the case of a cot, you may want to buy a new mattress. A good twin pram bought second-hand usually still has some resale value when you've finished with it. Second-hand clothes are often harsh to the touch, but can be fine.

The good news? You do not need:

- additional night attire for the babies
- cot bumpers (they look nice, but a baby can get trapped inside one, and later a more mobile infant can climb on to it and fall out of the cot)
- cot pillows (because of the risk of suffocation)
- special pram sheets (fold a cot sheet instead)
- Moses baskets or cribs (they are soon outgrown, and as you would have bought two, they are doubly extravagant).

· *Nappies* ·

Throw out or keep?

Disposable nappies are a great boon and are now made to fit almost all shapes and sizes of bottoms. Most mothers of twins go for disposables, but this depends on you and your lifestyle. Reusable nappies have also come on in leaps and bounds lately, and some are pre-shaped, which makes nappy-changing faster than with traditional 'terries'. Reusables aren't necessarily ecologically more sound since they have to be washed, using electricity and detergent. You may be able to get this done commercially instead of doing it yourself. Reusables are no better or worse for nappy rash than disposables, though they need changing a bit more often as they're usually less absorbent than modern disposables. Once you've bought them, they work out a little cheaper, but obviously they are going to be more time-consuming – a vital consideration with two or more babies.

You will need to splash out on about three dozen reusable nappies for twins. It sounds a lot, but some will be in soak. Use two nappy buckets if necessary rather than a single huge one, which can be back-breaking to handle when full.

If you take the disposable route, find a cash-and-carry to get a better price, or get nappies delivered to save time and energy. Many supermarkets do this. Some parents are concerned about the chemical content of disposables, especially the gels designed to draw moisture away from the baby's skin. All I can say is that I have never seen any adverse reactions to these, and there is no evidence of any toxic effect on a baby's testicles or any other organs either. With disposables, your main problem will be space in the bin, and with reusables it's going to be lack of time. Your call.

When to change?

Before a feed seems handy, in case the babies doze off while feeding, but this can delay – noisily – a hungry baby's feed. Besides, feeding tends to fill a nappy by reflex action, so all in all it is best to change a nappy after a feed unless it was already dirty or soaking wet. Keep nappy-changing gear both upstairs and downstairs to save you running up and down more than you have to.

· *Bathing* ·

You don't need to bath your twins every day. It can be a form of playtime for them and you, but there are less tiring ways of playing together. Besides, some young babies hate baths and are very vocal about getting the message across.

Newborn babies mainly get dirty at each end, so just keep their faces and nappy areas clean on a daily basis. Use warm water and cotton wool for 'topping and tailing'. You need only bath each baby on alternate days, unless you want to do it more often. (Incidentally, there is no need to change the water for each baby unless the first one opens his bowels in it, but that rarely happens). To save your back, use a stand for the bath, and don't carry around a full baby bath unless you really must.

· *Avenues of Help* ·

When work colleagues, friends or family ask what you would need as a present, ask for a contribution towards a night nurse for one night. When we had triplets, we booked a maternity nurse for eight weeks. She came on Monday, Tuesday and Wednesday nights and took over from 10 p.m. till 8 a.m., covering three feeds with the babies, and made all the bottles for the next day. We went to bed when she arrived. My husband covered the 3 a.m. feed on Friday and Saturday nights, and I did it on Thursday and Sunday nights. This kept us sane, as we knew for five nights of the week we would get sleep.

Apart from feeding and changing, there is bathing, washing, shopping, not to mention the rest of life . . . You need help. If this is your first pregnancy, you may be all at sea. If you already have children, you will have even more to do.

Many expectant mothers wait until after the birth to organise help, by which time they are surrounded by demanding babies and find it more difficult to make sensible arrangements. It's worth thinking ahead, ideally while still pregnant.

What you need depends on your circumstances. Who else is there around? Do you have other children? Will you be at work? Can you afford paid help? Have you a spare room?

The ideal helper is practical, willing, and reliable, not just someone who pops round every so often for cups of tea and coos over your little bundles.

- Your partner is the most obvious source of help (and moral support) in the first few days at home, especially if he takes paternity leave. During this special time, you can get to know your babies together and bond more closely as a couple, as well as doing chores in double-quick time. Even men who claim not to know one end of a baby from the other can turn out to be highly capable.
- Grandparents who live nearby can be worth their weight in gold. They will adore the grandchildren and boast about 'their' twins or triplets. However, if you have waited years to start your family, your parents may be elderly and less fit. They may also have old-fashioned ideas; even up-to-date tips may not be much use if they apply only to singletons.

- Neighbours and friends are useful if they have time to spare. The trouble is that they are often delighted to worship the babies but cannot make a regular commitment. You need 'do-ers' not 'see-ers'. If you have an acquaintance who can 'do' – or who has a teenaged son or daughter who is willing – consider paying them to put the arrangement on a business-like footing. They will be less likely to let you down.
- Volunteers from your local church or temple or other local groups may be happy to help. Or you could contact Home Start, a charity which has local networks of trained volunteers who help young families in their own home. Your health visitor, GP or midwife may also have ideas.

On the whole, there is little support for new mothers of multiples. Unless there are compelling reasons, Social Services have little to offer mothers of twins or triplets, but may be able to assist those with quads or quins. If you are offered a home help, establish what you will get when. It is pointless being told you can have two hours of home help a week, without knowing when those two hours will be; this sometimes happens.

Paid help

This includes:

- Maternity nurses: highly skilled (and highly paid) help for the first few weeks.
- Nannies: either untrained or fully qualified; can be daily or live-in. A qualified daily nanny is the most expensive, and an untrained – but experienced – person may be preferable, especially as she may do more housework (negotiate at interview). As a mother of twins, you do not usually want someone to enjoy the babies and leave you with the chores.

- Mother's helps: do not usually have sole charge of the children and are willing to do housework.
- Au pairs: very variable in skills and attitude. They should not have sole charge of very young babies, but can still be helpful if you have the space.

Help at night is a godsend, especially in the first three months, but it is worth remembering that a baby's cries often wake the mother and no one else!

One promising source of part-time help is a local college NNEB (Nursery Nurse Education Board) course. A student nanny on the final year of this course is often delighted to be involved with twins or triplets and may be able to put in a day a week for several months.

Whatever help you arrange, and whether or not she lives with you, as a parent you have to learn to make some space in your lives for her. This bit can take getting used to.

We couldn't have managed without Fran [au pair], but we really wished we didn't need her. It was my first pregnancy and we had intended to spend the first days and weeks as a family to enjoy that special time together. However, since our baby turned out to be triplets, this became an impossible dream.

· *Crying* ·

Your babies may not cry much, though mine certainly did. Fortunately, newborn twins rarely set each other off, though they do have similar needs at similar times. This is the essence of the challenge of caring for multiples. They will obviously cry together when they are hungry, tired or colicky at the same time. You will learn to anticipate some of their wants, which is where a routine really comes into its own. On the other hand, some mothers have found that when one baby is screaming for something, the other one is mercifully quiet.

Why are they crying?

Crying in stereo puts appalling pressure on a parent. What should you do first? Why are they crying, anyway? It could be:

- hunger – you will soon learn to distinguish this cry from the way it builds up in pitch
- discomfort or pain
- boredom – especially after four weeks of age
- a dirty nappy – possibly.

Are they ill? You should suspect this if one or other baby:

- is drowsy
- is unusually fractious
- is off his feed
- has a dry nappy when you would expect it to be wet (a sign of dehydration)
- has loose stools
- is snuffly
- has noisy or laboured breathing.

If any of these applies, or you are worried, check with your GP or health visitor without delay. Inevitably, there will be a false alarm or two, but most family doctors are happy to help as they know that new parents are anxious; most GPs are parents too. If, however, your doctor is not all that interested in young children (and everyone has different areas of expertise), consider changing your GP.

In time, you will learn to trust your instincts and will recognise what your babies need when they are crying.

Meanwhile, watch out for the danger signs mentioned. A digital thermometer, used under the baby's arm, can help you decide when an infant is ill. Although not infallible, it is more accurate than a heat-sensitive strip held to the forehead. It may surprise you to hear that a digital thermometer is also more reliable that the newer and pricier ear thermometer.

Colic

Regular crying, particularly in the evenings, can be colic, a poorly understood condition which usually starts at two weeks of age and disappears at three months. It is also known as 'evening colic' and 'three-month colic'. Nobody knows the cause, but it may be an extreme variant of normal crying. However, there's sometimes a link between colic and milk intolerance, so in severe cases it may be worth changing a baby's formula. Talk to your doctor first about this and other possible remedies. Otherwise, just cuddle and comfort your colicky baby. Babies should not be put to sleep on their fronts, but holding him on his stomach, for instance draped over your forearm, may relieve your baby's discomfort. However, two colicky babies could soon wear out your arms and your patience.

Coping with crying babies

If your babies are crying but you know they are not hungry, thirsty, bored or ill, you must get through this time as best you can. Fortunately, someone other than their mother usually finds it easier. One good way of defusing the situation is to collar someone into looking after the babies while you go and sit (or lie) down quietly out of earshot for half an hour.

You can also try playing them music – Mozart is popular with many babies, but so is any music they may have heard a lot before birth. The sound of a vacuum cleaner also soothes some crying babies.

Putting on some music and leaving the room can work wonders all round, but it requires a mother with an iron will. And first make sure your babies won't come to any harm unsupervised.

Many mothers cope with crying twins by bundling them into the pram and wheeling them round the block. Alternatively, you could try a drive in the car. If this does the trick, you can stop and read a book, or else come home and try to get them back in the house without waking them up.

Baby massage

Massage has been used on babies for generations, in countries all over the world, but it's a relatively new practice in this country. Massaging can help soothe a baby, relieve colic and crying, and may even boost the circulation and immune system. To a baby it's tangible evidence that you love him, and it can improve bonding. The technique is described in most baby-care books. With twins or more, the challenge is finding time to do it, but it can be very satisfying for you and your babies. Choose a time when your babies aren't sleepy or screaming, and make sure your hands are warm.

With our toddler tucked up in bed, massage time was our truly special time with our twin boys. It was in the evening after their baths, when my husband was home, and we'd take our boys on to our own bed with their towels. After even a quick bath you have to go slow with massage, and it helped relax babies, Mum and Dad after an always hectic day! Even five years on the boys occasionally ask for a massage after bath-time.

Dummies

With twins or more, a baby may have to wait about a great deal while you are changing, dressing or bathing another. Here dummies can be a real boon. Dummies can interfere with teeth and speech development, but if you use them only occasionally problems shouldn't arise. Besides, a baby usually gives up his dummy when he no longer needs it. It helps if you:

- restrict a dummy to indoor use only
- do not let a baby who can walk use one
- use the dummy not as a toy but as an aid to sanity
- stop offering one if the baby doesn't seek it.

Do keep dummies clean and sterilise them often (a spare set is a good idea). Never keep a dummy on a ribbon around a baby's neck: he shouldn't need a dummy constantly and, more importantly, a ribbon could strangle him.

Where to turn

If you have trouble coping with crying babies, don't be ashamed of asking for help. After all, many mothers of singletons need to and the challenges facing you are so much greater. Sharing your frustrations and difficulties, especially when your babies are very demanding, is not a sign of weakness, nor does it imply that you are a rotten parent. Tamba Twinline (see Resources, page 372) offers support and guidance to families of multiples, given by trained volunteers who are themselves parents of twins, triplets or more. Help is available in the evening and at weekends, times of greatest need, yet when professionals are often most difficult to contact.

· *Postnatal Depression* ·

What about that image of a joyous family, with you, the serenely competent mother, doubly happy and glowing with pride? Well, the answer is that nobody is that happy all the time. Some new mothers even find that, despite themselves, this special time is marred by feeling low.

In its various forms, postnatal depression affects roughly 10 per cent of new mothers, and it's said to be slightly more common in those with twins or more. Over a 12-year period, Australian research found mothers of twins to be both more anxious and more depressed postnatally than women with singletons. Several British studies also confirm that mothers of twins suffer more from fatigue, anxiety and emotional distress. Sometimes depression, especially in its milder forms, persists long after babyhood. Research shows that a slightly higher proportion of mothers with five-year-old twins are depressed.

At this point let me make two things clear: firstly, there's nothing intrinsically depressing about twins. They are lovely. It's the emotional, physical and financial challenges that can get you down. Secondly, the supposedly higher risk of postnatal depression may have a lot to do with sheer tiredness. At any rate, the twin mums who aren't depressed greatly outnumber the ones who are.

Symptoms and diagnosis

Should things not be going well for you, get the right help, especially if you:

- are crying more than usual
- feel hopeless
- get no pleasure at all from your babies
- are unable to laugh or enjoy yourself

- become very introspective
- feel indecisive
- suffer excess guilt
- go off your food (or, conversely, start comfort-eating)
- sleep badly (even when the babies are quiet).

Some women with postnatal depression suffer only mildly, while for a few it is a major hurdle, sometimes with serious consequences, including marital problems and even child abuse. That's why it's worth taking seriously.

Unfortunately it is sometimes hard for a woman or her family to recognise the symptoms for what they are. Tears, anxiety and indecision can be part of early life with a new baby anyway (the so-called 'three-day blues'). Some mothers do not share their thoughts, afraid perhaps of being thought incapable of coping, or they simply do not mention them to the GP at the right time.

> *It was towards the end of the consultation when I began to feel comfortable enough to tell the doctor how I felt (including the fact that actually I didn't need the Pill she'd just prescribed because I doubted I'd ever want sex again). But by then I'd got up and the doctor seemed to have mentally switched into a different gear. As far as she was concerned the consultation was over. It was another two weeks before I got around to telling her what I was going through.*

To spot postnatal depression sooner, especially in its milder forms, your midwife or health visitor may ask you to complete a short questionnaire at about six weeks after birth. The ten items of the Edinburgh Questionnaire ask a mother to assess how she has felt in the last seven days. It includes such items as: 'I have blamed myself unnecessarily when things went wrong.' The questionnaire can be a way of identifying the needs of some women who might not otherwise voice their concerns.

Causes

Acute mood swings ('three-day blues') are linked with wild hormonal fluctuations, but nobody is sure exactly what brings on the more lasting condition of postnatal depression. It can't just be hormones, because new fathers can also have typical symptoms. Postnatal depression may be an accentuated reaction to the stresses of new parenthood.

Treatment

Sometimes all a mother needs is practical and emotional support. This can come from family and helpers, or from talking things over with a health visitor, GP, midwife, or another experienced mother of twins.

A few women need more formal help from a counsellor, psychiatrist, psychologist or psychotherapist. Your GP can arrange this.

Anti-depressants can be very useful in some cases, and – contrary to popular perception – they are not habit-forming, unlike sedatives and sleeping pills. They don't work instantly, but they can make all the difference, probably because true depression has a biochemical element. The newer anti-depressants cause less drowsiness (you don't need to feel sleepier than you already are), but doctors often favour the older type if a woman is breast-feeding.

Dads may need to have their own feelings recognised too, and need time and support to adjust to their new role. I doubt enough is done for beleaguered fathers, but they too can ring Tamba Twinline.

Making things easier

You can't always help feeling low, but you can make positive improvements on several fronts to ease the first hectic few weeks:

1   Get into a routine as soon as you can. Mothers of singletons can afford a happy-go-lucky attitude to feeding, bathing and sleeping – they have much less to do! This is the single most useful piece of advice I can give, and it's a theme I'll come back to again in Chapter 6.

2   Use help available to achieve that end – a routine that makes some rest and recuperation possible.

3   Prioritise ruthlessly. You may have washed the net curtains on a weekly basis before or ironed tea-towels. Those days are gone. Prune housework back to the basic minimum needed for hygiene; anything more is a frill. Use your spare time for what matters: yourself and your immediate family.

4   Keep your own health up to par and get enough food, vitamins and rest (and do your postnatal exercises). YOU come first since so many others now depend totally on you.

5   Team up with other mothers of twins who understand your situation and can give you much-needed support. Friends with only one baby just can't know. Contact Tamba or your local twins group.

6   Manage stress. Mental and physical tension often go hand in hand, so learn a method of physical relaxation to help you let go. You can use an antenatal relaxation technique, or get a video, audio cassette or book from the public library.

7   Schedule a little 'me time' to do things you enjoy. This could be just a few minutes a day listening to your favourite music, but it is important to have time for yourself and also for you and your partner as a couple.

8   Get rid of guilt. New mums get a lot of well-meant advice but it's impossible to follow it all. You do not have to be perfect anyway. Being a 'good enough' parent is plenty.

9   Avoid isolation. It is harder for you to get out and about and your pre-twins life may seem a distant and unreal experience, but try to keep in touch with old friends and workmates. If you cannot get out much, use the phone and e-mail.

10   Everything may be rosy for you. I hope it is, but if you are feeling low, talk to someone. Telling your GP or health visitor why things are becoming too much can be the first vital step on the road to improvement.

Chapter Six

SURVIVING THE FIRST YEAR

How do mothers of singletons manage to fill their day?

It is natural to feel enormous pride in your babies, and besides, doesn't everyone keep saying how lucky you are to have twins? True, you are very lucky. But at the end of the day any parent has only two arms and one spine. Mothers of twins or more soon find that, although they get lots of admiring glances and appreciative remarks, there are few offers of practical help.

Babies usually learn to walk around the age of twelve months – some earlier, some a lot later. Because they are growing heavier but are still helpless, the first year brings huge logistic difficulties along with the delights. Obviously the more willing hands there are, the easier life is, but not everyone has able grandparents nearby or can afford paid help. Research confirms the suspicion that mothers of twins get out of the house much less often than mothers of singletons.

At home there is so much to do. A mum of twins can spend nearly twice as long on mundane chores related to the babies, which halves the time she can spend directly with them. To work out the time left for each of the twins, halve that again: each twin gets about a quarter of the attention a singleton has. So when can you find time to relate to your babies and savour the pleasures of being a twin mum?

Get into a routine as soon as you can. It will be based around your babies' sleep patterns. which could seem a bit haphazard at first. Learn to rest, either by snatching a siesta or just putting your feet up, when they're asleep.

· *Sleep* ·

Patterns of sleep vary from baby to baby. Babies under six months old could sleep 13–15 hours in every 24, but either or both of yours may need much less, and they may sleep at different times. Whatever their pattern, or lack of it, get your tiny tots used to falling asleep without holding, rocking, lulling or singing each baby to sleep. It's the thing you must do to establish good sleep habits.

Many things will help get your babies into a blissful routine and avert serious sleep problems:

- a room which is comfortable, being neither too cold nor too warm
- a regular bedtime
- a pleasant and predictable bedtime routine
- going in to check a crying baby but not picking him up
- night attire which is comfortable, without tight sleeves, constricting wristbands, and so on
- night-lights or, paradoxically, dark curtains/curtain lining
- dummies
- keeping any night-feeds and nappy changes as brief and business-like as possible
- learning to relax yourself.

Where should your babies sleep? For the first six months, in the same room as you if possible. Later, probably in another room. Some multiples disturb each other, but many gain satisfaction from being together in the same room. There are no fixed rules, and you will soon know what's best for your babies.

Co-bedding: twins sleeping together

Many parents 'co-bed' their twins in the first month of life, and some still do at three months. A lot depends on what was started in hospital. Do twins disturb each other when they're in the same cot? Dr Helen Ball from the University of Durham carried out extensive research into co-bedding and concluded that twins sleeping in close proximity to each other don't wake more often. Their sleep–waking patterns are more similar, though, which parents can find helpful. However, the biggest advantage is that you only need one cot for the time being, and that may mean that you can keep them in your bedroom even if you don't have space for two cots. A big question is whether co-bedding could prevent cot death (sudden infant death syndrome or SIDS). Probably not: it's the presence of you or another adult that's linked with a reduction in cot death.

Co-sleeping: twins in your bed

It's hard to be sure of the right answers here as the research hasn't been done. Even with singletons, the practice is controversial, with some experts suggesting that sudden infant death syndrome (SIDS) might be more common when a baby shares a parent's bed (or sofa). Whether you can safely take a baby to bed with you is uncertain. You definitely shouldn't if you or your partner is a smoker, has been drinking alcohol, takes any drugs or medication that can make you drowsy, or is feeling very tired. For more on SIDS, see the Appendix.

With twins, added problems might include a higher risk of overheating. If you decide to take your babies to bed with you, it's especially important to keep blankets lightweight and avoid duvets and pillows. There's also the danger of one or other baby tumbling out of bed. Some parents take their twins to bed on a double mattress on the floor. It's difficult to give a verdict on this because there's just not enough evidence to go on.

Sleep problems

Soon after the age of six months, babies acquire the ability to stay awake deliberately (and apparently indefinitely) even when they, and you, are worn out. They can of course also be kept awake by discomfort, hunger, illness or teething, causes which you may need to consider and rule out.

In many ways, sleepless twins differ little from sleepless singletons, but their impact is greater because your days are more demanding. It is hard to enjoy your twins if they wake you relentlessly night after night. It can also be a distinct drain on relationships within the family, for instance if you and your partner have agreed between you that you must bear the brunt of night-time duties so that he can be refreshed enough to function at the office.

It is often said that nobody ever died from lack of sleep, but psychologists in industry question this old saw. In everyday life, lack of sleep can lead to constant tiredness and symptoms of depression, and can seriously reduce effectiveness at home or at work.

If sleeplessness causes problems, it helps to:

- read the Tamba leaflet on sleeping problems in multiples (which also covers toddlers and older children)
- talk over your difficulties with your health visitor
- contact Twinline or CRY-SIS (see Resources, pages 372 and 373).

There are several tried and tested approaches for established sleeping problems. One, sometimes called the checking method, is to keep checking but not picking up a crying baby. Go to your child when he cries and let him know you are nearby. Instead of lifting him, however, simply tuck him in or pat him, then say goodnight and leave. He may wail again (if he has stopped at all), but do not return to him for three to five minutes. Use a watch to time yourself, as it will seem endless. Gradually lengthen the time between checks. This firm approach is also called the controlled crying method and is often recommended by health visitors and many other childcare experts. It may sound cruel, but you are not being unkind if you have already established there is nothing physically wrong. Many parents are thrilled by how well it works, and it sometimes does the trick within a week or so. Others need longer. It is important to be consistent and confident, and of course to get the support of your partner too.

Withholding night-time drinks may help. Many young children who wake in the night are offered a beverage to settle them. If you gradually withdraw (for instance by diluting with water) the night-time drinks, they may become too unexciting to bother with, and there is therefore less of an incentive to clamour for one. Water is also better for young teeth: even pure fruit juices can rot a youngster's teeth.

If your babies seem to rouse each other, or perhaps one consistently wakes his twin, it may be a good idea to separate them at night, at least temporarily, if you can.

You will almost certainly succeed with one of these methods, or one of the other ideas from Tamba. If not, talk to your health visitor again.

· *Getting Out of the House* ·

With two or more babies, even the simplest outing is like a military campaign. And watch out for action from the rear. Just when they've been fed, changed, dressed and popped into their buggy (you have thought ahead and packed nappy-changing gear and their next feeds), and you have your hand on the front door to open it, one of them decides to fill his nappy. You get him out and change him again, by which time his twin is screaming with impatience. Don't get discouraged, as a little forward planning can work wonders.

I got it down to such a fine art that my friends would marvel. How was it that I managed to mobilise my two faster than they did their singletons?

Public transport

Many twin mums don't have the use of a car in the day. Although trains and undergrounds may not be too awful with a buggy if you can avoid stations with stairs, buses are often impossible for an unaided parent of multiples. You can sometimes manage twins in two slings, or one in a sling and the other in a buggy, but soon your back will let you know it is too much. If you have any choice in the matter, minimise these trips, and when you must go, take another adult with you.

Shopping

When the babies are in a pram or buggy, you can sometimes go round the supermarket with it, but once they sit up well unaided, a supermarket trolley made for twins is best, if available. Always use a harness. Mothers of triplets or more suggest leaving at least one baby at home with someone rather than attempting shopping trips with the whole mob. Even better, shop by phone or on the internet, and save your energies for more pleasant outings.

Making outings easier

- Keep the nappy-changing bag at the ready by the front door.

- Take toys along to allay boredom. Attaching toys to the buggy avoids too many losses. A couple of extra playthings hidden away in a bag can be handy if your outing is longer than planned.
- If bottle-feeding, have feeds ready in the fridge so that you don't come home with two starving babies and find nothing to give them.
- An extra feed in the changing bag is a good idea too.

Clinic visits

Mothers with twins and triplets weigh their babies less often than those with singletons, not because they need it less, but because it is such a hassle getting to the clinic. Transporting them there, undressing them, dressing them again and maybe consoling them after a jab can all seem too much.

- Health visitors may not have experience of multiples, so tell yours how she can help in practical ways. She could hold one of the babies for you, or arrange to weigh them and immunise them at home.
- Take along a friend when you go to the clinic if you can. Otherwise a receptionist may be free to assist.
- Prams are often forbidden inside the clinic, but you can ask. Once staff appreciate the problems, they may be happy to make an exception.
- You could adopt a tip from Tamba that several mothers find helpful: weigh each baby fully clothed, then subtract the weight of identical clothes you have put in the changing bag just for this purpose.

· *Coping at Home in the First Year* ·

The only point of having baby equipment is to make life safer for your babies and easier for you. So how best to use what is available?

Play-pens

You can do without a play-pen, but they're useful for safety if nothing else. Your babies can play in one reasonably unmolested if you have a jealous toddler. You can pop them in the play-pen when you answer the door or go to the loo, and it is also handy in the garden. A play-pen is a good place for an impromptu nap, too.

A second-hand play-pen is usually fine, but good solid construction is vital since two babies give it twice as much of a battering. It is tempting to use it a lot if you have multiples, as many mothers admit, but try not to overdo it. No matter how many toys they have with them, babies don't benefit from long hours in a play-pen because they can't get personal attention or explore the wider world. Besides, if you keep dumping them in the play-pen they will begin to hate it.

Highchairs

You need highchairs some time in the first year, usually between five and eight months, when your twins sit up to eat. Always use a proper harness as well. Supervise your babies even when eating finger-food: they can choke on a rusk. They also tend to pinch each other's food when they can reach it! Folding highchairs obviously save space.

Highchairs are widely available in family restaurants, but if you need three or more, it is wise to ring first and request them.

There are portable seats that turn chairs into highchairs, as well as an ingenious cloth harness called a Tam-Sit that can do a similar job. This is useful when travelling.

Baby-bouncers, baby-gyms, etc.

These are seats that hang from a frame or doorway in which your baby bounces up and down. The fun tends to last only a few minutes per session, so most mothers of twins cannot be bothered with them. However, the entertainment lasts much longer if you have two baby-bouncers, and two door frames close together, so that the babies can see each other. Some swings on a frame are battery-operated, and mums who've used them with their twins say they're wonderful.

Baby-walkers

You might think these little seats on wheels are great fun, but they have a lot of drawbacks. Any child left on the floor gets his hands and feet run over, so if you have twins, you need two walkers, or none. With two or three baby-walkers whizzing around, your living room becomes a fairground complete with dodgems. More importantly, baby-walkers are dangerous because they can tip up easily. Near the top of the stairs they are lethal. Walkers are the most common piece of home equipment involved in baby and child accidents. Even if you supervise very closely and avoid mishaps, excessive use may be damaging and could delay learning to walk.

Keeping an eye on your babies

Babies usually crawl from about seven or eight months, and stand at eight to 10 months, but even before this they can get into serious trouble. Anything small finds its way into little mouths, so watch out for things such as beads, buttons, small batteries (especially harmful if swallowed) and an older sibling's Lego. The same applies to singleton babies, but when you have two or more you really need to be on the ball.

As soon as your babies are a couple of months old, start assessing potential dangers. Try to size up your home from their point of view and remove or alter any hazards. You can get lots of tips and advice from RoSPA (Royal Society for the Prevention of Accidents) and CAPT (Child Accident Prevention Trust) (see Resources, pages 375 and 373).

However hard you try, a totally childproof home does not exist, and would probably be very dull if it did. At this stage you need to watch over your twins practically all the time. Bathtime is particularly dangerous, so never leave one or more babies alone in any bath. They can drown in less than 2.5 cm (an inch) of water: babies have been known to die in the fluid at the bottom of a nappy bucket. As for your own ablutions, you may have company, in the form of two little faces peering at you over the edge of the tub.

Safety gates are almost essential, and you could need them for a long time. The fixed type, screwed into the wall, is more bother but much sturdier and especially useful at the top of the stairs. You need a gate at the bottom of the stairs too. It can also be handy to have a movable gate to use across doorways as needed, for instance to keep your babies out of the kitchen. Even here you may prefer a fixed gate: working as a team, two or more babies can pull down a gate that totally defeats a singleton.

· *Playing* ·

Young babies need to play with things. The question is, how many of what should you buy? You may want two of some things, like rattles, but these needn't be identical. And you don't have to duplicate everything. You need only one of some bigger items.

Toys can be very expensive, which is where toy libraries come in. Remember too that egg cartons, cotton reels, etc, are free and can be playthings too.

Talking and eye contact are the best entertainment of all,

especially for multiples, and cost only time. Babies enjoy (and learn from) being smiled at, tickled, held, stroked, sung to, talked to and read to, long before they can speak. Many mothers play spontaneously with their babies, though some are self-conscious or find it difficult.

It really doesn't matter whether you make a fool of yourself in front of your babies or read to them from *The Times*, as a friend of mine did. Your attention is all-important, particularly when provided on an individual basis for each baby, even if only for a few minutes at a time. If you can't manage this, play with your babies together, but try to make eye contact with each in turn.

· *Weaning* ·

Your babies will be ready for solids between four and six months of age (WHO recommendations are that babies should be fed breast-milk alone for the first six months, but most paediatricians agree that this policy is more suited to developing countries than the western world). This is only an approximate guide, because smaller babies usually need solids later than larger ones. A clue that a baby needs solids is when he reverts to night feeds a few weeks after you thought he'd given them up for good.

In general, it is best to try both or all your babies on solids at the same time, unless they are very different in size. Bear in mind, though, that one may take to solid food first.

The principles of starting solids are just the same as for a single baby, but the mess is greater. If you haven't had a baby before, you may be shocked by how much food ends up on the outside of the babies.

• Sit the babies in bouncing cradles or car seats to start with (or in a buggy if you are out), moving on to highchairs as they become better at sitting up.

- Don't use your sitting room for meals if you can help it. The kitchen is ideal if you have the space. Spread newspapers out on the floor beneath the babies. You can use plastic sheeting, but it is tedious to wipe it every time; newspaper can be thrown away after each meal.

- Put on the answering machine if you have one.

- Use plastic bibs with a pelican-type trough. At the end of the meal just tip out the slops. These bibs don't last for ever, so buy new ones as necessary.

- In warm weather, the babies can be stripped down to nappy and vest to avoid unnecessary laundering.

- Multiples tend to share germs, so, unless there are compelling medical reasons, use one spoon and one bowl for both (or all) babies. Feed a spoonful to each in turn, stopping only to fill up the spoon. You will find that once they get the hang of it, they sit up with their mouths permanently open like tiny birds and you will hardly be able to keep up with demand. This looks very cute but can be noisy.

- So that they still grasp the idea of cutlery, you can give each baby a spare plastic spoon to hold, wave about, bash against the highchair, hit his brother with, etc.

- Take different tastes in your stride. Unless there are definite allergies, they should still be offered the same foods (catering now for their preferences could be troublesome later). If you don't go to a lot of trouble to prepare tasty meals, you will be less upset when they reject them.

- Ice-cube trays are often suggested for freezing portions of home-prepared baby food, but empty yoghurt pots, cottage cheese containers, etc. are a better size with twins or more.

- Finger-foods come into their own from about six or seven months and your babies may have fun trying to feed each other. This is also a time when they will want to try feeding themselves – messy but essential. The temptation with multiples is to spoon-feed them for as long as possible to minimise chaos and save time, but they must be allowed to learn, even if they use yoghurt as fingerpaint and stewed fruit as a face-pack. You will have many more problems later if you don't let them.

- If you are eating at the same time, which becomes possible once the babies get to finger-foods, try to set a good example. With luck, they might just copy you. As they get older, it becomes more important to take your meals with them.

- Training them to sit still for meals even without a highchair is quite easy towards the end of the first year. Sit them on a blanket or sheet. Just remove the food if they get up. Later, they may even eat their sandwiches at picnics without crawling away mid-meal.

- In the early days, you will be finishing off each session of solids with a bottle (or breast), but try to get your babies on to cups or drinkers when you can. Most babies go through a stage at about six months when they really take to a beaker, which is much better for them: drinks from bottles are more likely to damage developing teeth.

- Sometimes one baby will give up the breast or bottle first, and the other follows within a few weeks. This is completely normal. Meanwhile, enjoy the closeness of feeding just one.

· *When They are Ill* ·

Minor illnesses are common with any under-fives. Infections are even more common in the first few months of a premature baby's life.

Twins don't necessarily get ill simultaneously, but they sometimes do. When one or other is unwell, keeping both of them happy becomes a juggling act, especially if you have to carry the sick one around most of the time. Under these circumstances the well one may become particularly demanding. On the other hand, many mothers find that, thankfully, the opposite happens: the healthy one is content to make do with very little from you while his twin is ill.

With triplets or more, you'll feel very stretched during even minor illnesses. Common infections can turn family life upside down, especially with stomach upsets or diarrhoea. Episodes like this, say many mums of triplets, are the lowest points of their first year. Any help with chores or one of the babies is more than welcome. Now is the time to take up any offers you were rash enough to decline when all was well.

A fractious youngster is much happier and easier to handle once any fever is controlled, so do give paracetamol syrup or whatever your doctor has recommended for fever. Make sure he gets enough fluid to drink – you may have to tempt him often – and don't overwrap a sick baby. Some remedies, like steam inhalations, become impossible with more than one small child.

Unless they are very ill, many sick babies can still go out in a pram or buggy, even if grandparents are horrified by this new-fangled practice. Most babies appreciate a change of scene. If you really are confined to the house, use different rooms at various times of the day if you can.

When you need a doctor, your thoughts may turn to house calls. There are times when it's impossible to get to the surgery, so ask for a visit if you really need one. However, you can get medical attention a lot quicker if you can manage to get to the surgery. Make sure the receptionist knows you have twins, to minimise any waiting. A receptionist may even be able to hold one of your babies. Insist on separate appointments for each baby, and talk about each separately. Otherwise you and your doctor will get hopelessly muddled.

Each baby should also have his own medicines. Babies

shouldn't share prescriptions, only paracetamol and over-the-counter medicines. Keep a diary to log medications you give them, temperature readings, and so on.

Make sure your twins never share medical records or a child health book. Treat each one as completely separate; even identicals don't always have the same allergies, for instance.

Sometimes a GP will press for hospital admission for a condition that perhaps could be treated at home in a singleton. It is challenging to look after a very poorly baby when you have others to care for too, but discuss this with your doctor.

If one of your babies has to go into hospital, you must decide whether to take the other one too. The answer is probably no, unless you are breast-feeding or the babies are very small, or, perhaps as a single parent, you have no option. If your babies have never been apart, you may also want to have both admitted, to save added trauma for both babies. Hospitals should be flexible about multiples but they're not always.

Jack developed an emergency inguinal hernia at eight weeks old. He was admitted for surgery, but as I was breast-feeding both boys we all had to stay for three days. A week later, the story was repeated with Patrick, and two weeks later Patrick again developed a hernia on his other side. Nursing staff resented an extra 'well' baby on the ward, so gave me little or no help even with whichever boy was ill. Less than a month later, Jack was admitted with bronchiolitis. As I couldn't face the lack of support, I didn't stay with him, and I insisted on taking him home the next day.

Nowadays, hospitals are used to mums or dads staying the night with their baby. In fact, you may be relied on to provide much of the care. This will do a lot for your sick baby, though it is likely to exhaust you further. A grandparent who can stay and give you a hand when you get home is a great help.

When one twin is ill, you may worry about the other baby developing the same condition. This can obviously happen with infectious illnesses, and there's not much you can do about it. They usually share the same germs anyway, so it's pointless going to elaborate lengths to keep them apart or sterilise more things than usual. Sometimes twins also get the same non-infectious diseases, like an inguinal hernia.

· *Making Life Easier* ·

The first year can be a strain. Your partner will have had to pitch in a lot, helping to care for the babies, doing domestic chores, giving you support, and carrying on with his own work, perhaps on little sleep. Meanwhile, older siblings' lives will have changed too (a topic covered in Chapter 9).

Normal family activities seem to have been abandoned, or exchanged for a never-ending round of chores. If you have help at home, you may have more time for each other and the children, at the expense of less privacy.

Parents of triplets or more have a particularly hard time. The National Study of Triplets and Higher Order Births confirms that many triplet mothers have health problems in the first year, as do some of their partners. Many parents have found their relationship strengthened, but for some couples caring for multiples has the opposite result.

You've put that Caribbean holiday on hold. For now, just getting out of the house seems an achievement. Compared with your previous existence, the rare outings you get appear very dull, but I promise you it will improve. Understand that this is a new phase of your life. It will be better and richer, but for now it is a period of transition and that is always hard, especially if you're tired.

Many twin mums later regret having spent so much time

and energy on drudgery and chores in the first 12 months instead of being with the babies and enjoying them. You can make it easier on yourself by re-examining your priorities and by realising before it is too late that time is precious.

Get into a routine you can live with. The sooner your babies' habits are synchronised and simplified, the better. You still don't have to give them all daily baths until they're on solids and crawling. Ironing is also superfluous too (and dangerous with babies around).

Make a point of playing with your babies and giving them attention. Go out regularly, for instance to toddler groups, no matter how hard it is. Once you escape from siege conditions, you will all benefit from socialising. Many mums say a daily outing keeps them sane.

Get help if you can. Perhaps a friend's au pair, or a neighbour's teenaged daughter, could spare a few hours a week. She could look after a baby for an hour or so, do the shopping or perhaps give an older sibling his own outing.

If you are back at work, make sure your child-carer contributes to the domestic chores. If your babies go to a child-minder, can you enlist some other help with housework or washing? Note that a child-minder for two babies can work out expensive; you may be better off with someone who comes to your house. It is normal for nannies to do the children's washing and keep their rooms clean, but could she also wash the kitchen floor? Negotiate at the outset. Unqualified nannies are often more flexible on this, and not necessarily less experienced.

Take the long view. If you've got this far, you are probably doing well. There will be good days and less good days, but there is no need to punish yourself when you don't get things quite right. You can only do so much.

If you can afford it, consider a family holiday soon. Your twins probably aren't mobile yet and may be happy sitting in a pushchair for a while. Because they are under two years old, you may get some reasonably priced deals. You'll probably have most fun if you try not to be too ambitious.

Make some time for yourself and your partner. However remote the future seems now, your children will eventually grow up and then where will you be?

· *The Light at the End of the Tunnel* ·

Most available research – and advice – on rearing twins concentrates on the hardships and difficulties of having more than one child at a time. There is no doubt this first year is a challenge, which makes it all the more necessary to give some thought to the joys of multiples – and there are plenty of those, believe me.

> *Whenever I felt low in the first few months, I'd bundle my babies into their huge pram, which was the size of a skip, and head for the streets where I'd be bound to get gasps of admiration from total strangers.*

> *I'd come home from work and they'd cling to me like limpets, one on each of my legs. It certainly makes you feel wanted.*

> *After bathtime, they'd clamber all over me with their little pink bodies still wet and glistening from the bath, and smelling fantastic. I'll never forget that baby smell.*

> *If I have been away for a morning, the inexplicable joy of three little faces lighting up when they catch sight of you is amazing.*

The following list incorporates views from parents as well as findings from projects carried out by Dr Herbert Collier of Phoenix, Arizona, who, unusually for a researcher, decided to highlight the pleasures of having twins.

- Twins (and more) are often amazingly cute-looking and stay that way much longer than most singletons. This is one reason why they attract so much attention, which many parents enjoy.
- It is fun to watch their individual personalities develop, at least twice as fascinating as with a singleton.
- Watching them interact is brilliant. Even at this tender age, they smile and gurgle at each other and appear to have a tacit understanding.
- Soon you may also notice a special bond developing between the twins. Young twins sometimes learn to share things such as drinks, biscuits and toys quite spontaneously (however, don't bank on it).
- Even when they are not particularly close, twins have someone else to share life's joys and problems with and are a comfort to each other.
- Many parents of multiples say that, however shocked they were when they received the news, they somehow feel special, lucky or blessed.
- Dads of twins often benefit from being far more involved in the day-to-day care of the children than they would have been with a singleton.
- You get double the joy, love, and cuddles (often from both at the same time).
- You do have to re-focus your life, but this is often all to the good and can be an enriching experience which brings new friends and a new emphasis.
- Once they get to the end of the first year, many mothers feel an intense sense of achievement and elation. If you can manage twins, you can manage almost anything.

Chapter Seven

IDENTITY AND INDIVIDUALITY

You're just two halves of the same person.

If you think that was a remark from someone who knows nothing about twins, you're in for a shock. It came from a person who really should know better: a secondary school teacher who is a parent of multiples.

Those who remember Alice's adventures through the looking-glass will know that Tweedledum and Tweedledee could be distinguished only by the words Dum and Dee on their collars. They agreed to have a battle – not unusual for young twins. Tweedledum said Tweedledee had spoilt his nice new rattle. Perhaps he was just laying the blame for the damage on his twin, or perhaps it was actually Tweedledum who had broken Tweedledee's rattle. Who knows whether Lewis Carroll would have even written about them had they not been so identical in every way.

Twins, triplets or more are of course individuals. Even identical twins aren't truly identical, as I've explained in Chapter 1. But I think something often happens when people come across many same-sex twins. Somewhere inside the brain, a twin-switch seems to flip on. From then on, they find they can't even tell apart twins who are very different to look at. They even stop trying. I know my own twin-switch was in the on position whenever I saw a particular pair of twins at playgroup. They were totally unalike, Claire being tall and well built, while Louise was thin and small, yet along with many other adults I had a persistent mental block which prevented me from ever addressing them correctly.

Early on in life, identical twins can have trouble telling each other apart. When you have grown alongside someone else all along, it can be hard to know what is you and what isn't. The classical example is the identical twin looking into a mirror: is the image himself or his twin? If he sucks a thumb, is it his own or his brother's?

> *Sometimes Alex gets confused in front of the mirror. He doesn't seem to know who the reflection is, or who he is. The other day he and Kim were both looking in the mirror, and the only way he could resolve this question was to bite his brother. Kim and his reflection cried, and Alex's problem was solved.*

Twins and their parents evolve ways of making distinctions. Perhaps this is why twins often seem to allot each other different roles, so that they complement each other. At its most obvious, one starts a sentence and the other finishes it. One may make friends while the other remains in the background. One may try new things, whereas his twin does not, and so on. The French psychologist Professor René Zazzo calls this division of labour between twins 'the couple effect'.

The 'couple effect' can even mask or obscure genetic similarities. Research shows that identical twins brought up together tend to be less alike than identicals brought up apart. Why? Perhaps it is because that's how the twins strive to be. Of course, parents influence their children profoundly: adults probably both create and respond to any differences the children show. Many parents cherish and encourage their twins' dissimilarities. One could call these 'splitters'. There are also 'lumpers', parents who value their children's twin-ness above their other characteristics and tend to treat them as one unit.

Every human being needs a sense of self. While your

twins are growing up and learning to function independently of you, they have the extra task of growing away from each other and developing this sense of self. This process, called individuation, means becoming a complete person, with an ability to form functional relationships with others. Dealing with twins as one unit interferes with this process and can cause long-term distress (a topic explored in Chapter 16).

As parents we all want our children to grow up to be functional adults. The sooner you start helping them become individuals, the better. If your twins or triplets are already a year old, it is relatively late to begin, but there's still everything left to play for.

By-products of promoting your multiples' separate identities

Nurturing your children's individuality has many other benefits along the way. It helps build their social skills. Since children learn language and speech by example, their communication skills will also improve. Many scuffles between twins are ploys for attention. Treating your twins as individuals can make them less competitive and less likely to fight. It could improve their behaviour, or at least make it easier for a parent to deal with lapses. You will certainly find parenting more satisfying if you relate to each twin as an individual. Your twins' school careers may also be easier in terms of both schoolwork and social development. Treating your children as individuals will also make adolescence less difficult. Not easier, just less difficult. Adolescence is a tough time, but those twins who are treated as separate beings tend to have more confidence (see Chapter 14).

Psychologist Sara Smilanski has studied how twins become individuals, and used what she called an individuation score as a mark of self-confidence. She found that, between the ages of six and eight years, single-born children were the most strongly individual, as you'd expect. Non-identical (dizygotic or DZ, see pages 16–19) twins were somewhat less individual, while identical (monozygotic or MZ) twins the least. Between ages nine and 10, the non-identical twins were almost as self-confident as singletons, but the identical twins lagged behind, and this difference persisted into the teen years.

· *Clothes* ·

Sure, clothes are superficial, but the fact is that people do judge others by appearance, and parents of twins are no exception. To relate to each twin (or triplet) in his own right, it's essential to be able to tell them apart in the first place. Should you dress twin babies alike? Twins or more look sweet dressed identically and fit in with most people's concept of 'twin-ness'. In the very early days, it doesn't much matter what they wear as long as you (or anyone else looking after them) can distinguish them easily. This is important on safety grounds: twins have ended up with a double dose of antibiotics because their child-minders could not tell them apart.

But it's best not to do this for long. Infant twins themselves soon notice what they are wearing. Even as early as nine months, they can get upset if they're usually dressed alike and then you suddenly clothe them differently.

There's even research showing that twins aged two to four who are dressed alike may have more behaviour problems and score less well in language tests. There are many possible reasons why this might be, but it's certainly food for thought.

The same outfits in different colours are a cute way to dress multiples, but sticking too rigidly to colour codes can store up trouble for later on. Some twins may later reject their school uniform or PE bag in house colours on the grounds that it is not 'their' colour.

Another option is to dress them in similar colours but different styles. This can be especially attractive on young triplets and boy-girl pairs, who may not otherwise look much like multiples. Alternatively, you could forget about matching outfits altogether, which is obviously a lot easier because you can put them in whatever comes to hand in the morning.

You will inevitably be given sets of identical clothes for your babies, at least in the very early days. Nevertheless, you need not dress them the same: one baby can have, say, both turquoise sleep-suits while his brother has the two yellow ones.

· *Twin-ness* ·

I love it when my girls look the same.

What about your own feelings? Most people have only one baby at a time, and it's normal to cherish and even brag about your babies being twins. We parents have worked hard for it! You can however still revel in their twin-ness, and in your status as a parent of twins, while helping each of your babies achieve his own unique potential.

Time is your greatest enemy. It's expedient to lump twins or triplets together, to talk to them at the same time and to treat them generally as one unit. A child-minder once told me that caring for eight-month-old twins was no different from looking after one baby. While I was glad she felt that competent, it made me look around for some other arrangement.

It takes time to nurture children as individuals. Your schedule is already full, what with the feeding, the endless washing, and maybe going to work. But I like to think we mums and dads of multiples are equal to the special mission entrusted to us.

If you are still expecting

Before they are born, prepare the rest of the family for the arrival not just of twins, but of two little individuals. Although grandparents will naturally be thrilled, the older generation may be more likely to be 'lumpers'. Get them used to the idea of, say, minding one twin at a time, which is easier for them anyway.

When you're organising your support systems, make sure your arrangements will allow your babies to be treated as individuals as much as possible. You may need to spell this out to any home help or au pair you have, for instance.

Choice of names is very important, a topic covered in Chapter 2.

After they are born

Learn pronto how to tell them apart. Make frequent eye-contact, no matter how bleary-eyed you may be from lack of sleep, and learn to relate to each baby separately.

Encourage absolutely everyone to use their names from the start. Sometimes it's tempting to use collective nouns for your children (for example, twins, boys, gang, mob, twiglets, dynamic duo, awesome foursome), but for their sakes keep this to a minimum. Nobody should be allowed to call them 'the twins' when talking to them (as opposed to talking about them).

This isn't always as straightforward as it seems. Professor René Zazzo found that 10 per cent of parents couldn't recall which baby had originally been given which name! Also, even when you know perfectly well who is who, you can still say the wrong word when you are in a hurry (just as you can occasionally slip up and use a son's name when addressing your partner).

Here's what Samuel Clemens (Mark Twain) had to say about the matter:

> *My twin and I got mixed up in the bath-tub when we were two weeks old and one of us was drowned, but we didn't know which. Some say it was Bill, some say it was me. One of us had a peculiar mark – a large hole on the back of his left hand, but that was me. That was the one that was drowned.*

At some point in the first year, you and your partner will probably realise how different your twins are in personality, even if they look like two peas in a pod. Dissimilarities are noticeable from the word go:

> *Both had an untraumatic birth – I had a caesarean without going into labour – and both weighed exactly the same. Alistair was the placid one from the first day, but Gareth would startle very easily, especially if anyone brushed against his hospital cot and made it swing. It only swung by a few degrees but he seemed to hate it and his limbs would jerk out. Alistair was in a type of cot that didn't move at all, so I swapped them round. Gareth settled, and the swinging cot never bothered Alistair at all.*

It's all too easy for parents of twins to focus on differences and magnify them. We want our children to be individuals, and perhaps it is easier to relate to them once we establish who is 'the quiet one', 'the smiley one', 'the greedy one', or whatever. These tags may be real enough at the time, even helpful in the short term, but often they are merely temporary. As soon as you have decided who the naughty one is and who the good one is, your youngsters will reverse roles, just to keep you on your toes.

> *For several weeks, Amanda was a sweet-natured toddler and butter wouldn't melt in her mouth. Zoe, meanwhile, would*

grizzle and grump. But, lo and behold, for no reason at all they suddenly swapped and now Amanda behaved as if she had the devil in her.

Nobody really knows why this 'see-sawing' happens, but it's well known with multiples. The challenge facing parents is how to nurture individuality without using divisive labels.

As they grow up

Using the right names is a good start, but helping individuality ultimately depends on giving individual attention. Whenever you can, talk to each child separately rather than addressing them collectively. Try your best to use their individual names, even if it is only to say, 'Toby, leave that alone.' If both your children are present, use that child's name at the beginning of the sentence so he knows right away that you're talking to him.

It is an effort to repeat yourself for each twin or triplet, and you will inevitably end up saying such things as 'Look, a tree' rather more times than the average parent. It is worth it, however.

Some twins get confused between their name and their twin's. If this happens a lot, get the child who's being addressed to tap himself on the chest when you speak his name, and perhaps also point to his twin when you use his twin's name.

Multiples develop along different lines from singletons. At around 10 months they are very aware of each other. They babble together and may even comfort each other when upset. From 12 or 13 months they can play together, which is much earlier than single-born children play with others. When they play, they also copy each other. It helps if you also play with one child at a time occasionally. Read to each twin separately if you can, for instance at bedtime.

Bedtime stories are a good way of winding down active kids and getting them in the mood for sleep. But if you start reading to one while the other plays on the floor, you could soon find yourselves disturbed and interrupted. The ideal is to read to each child individually with the other one in another room, perhaps getting a story from your partner, but few twins and even fewer triplets have this luxury. However, you may be able to do this at weekends. During the week the children can share one story. Reading to them, whether separately or together, is a precious time for many parents, and if you can't manage separate sessions with each, so be it.

At this stage they should definitely have their own clothes. There are more safety issues now (see Chapter 8), and the more they do out of doors, the more important this is.

Each twin will value his own territory. They may share a bedroom but you could try to arrange some private play-space or shelves.

My girls each had her own special painting near her bed, done by their aunt who is an artist and quilt-maker. Each picture incorporated a fancy inital letter, A for Anna and R for Rebecca.

Each child could have his own toy-box and toys, except for building blocks, perhaps, and other really big items which are shared.

When you take photos and videos, as you are bound to, make sure you label them in some way so you can tell later which child is which. It's sad to look at family snaps in years to come and find that neither you nor the children knows who's in the picture. Take some photos of each twin on his own too.

Going to parties is a big part of childhood, with celebrations becoming more elaborate all the time. If both your children are invited, a discreet word with the birthday child's parents should ensure that each gets his own invitation and party bag. It's nice for each of your twins to reply separately to the invite, and to take separate presents to the party (they needn't be more expensive than one gift).

I've concentrated on things, but individuality is more about opportunities. Twins and other multiples are poor in opportunities to gain independence and self-esteem. There are practical limitations on their explorations, for a start. In the home, there's a risk of accidents if two, three or four babies crawl around the house, because you can't watch over all of them. In the park it's much the same story. A singleton may toddle off to explore, pursued by his relaxed, laughing mum who knows she'll easily catch up with him when she needs to. With twins, they often go off in different directions. Mum is in pursuit but she isn't laughing. She's tearing her hair out and screaming her head off. If she doesn't get both of them back quick, someone's bound to get run over . . . It's a lot less trouble to keep them in the buggy next time.

Messy play is also more difficult with multiples, as is learning to feed themselves. By 18 months, a toddler uses a spoon with confidence, though not necessarily with accuracy. Multiples too need to learn to eat independently, despite the time this can take.

By his second or third birthday, a child should be at least partly dressing himself, but with twins and a busy life it's easier for mums to carry on dressing their toddlers. Each one needs to learn to dress, as well as acquire other life-skills like toileting and hand-washing. Because twins can work as a team, you may not notice that only one of them does certain tasks. One mother didn't realise until her twin boys went to university that only one of them ever made breakfast at home for the both of them.

Most of all, twins lack solitude. There's no such thing as doing a puzzle on his own, because it won't be long before the other twin muscles in. Building a tower of bricks is fun, until your twin sabotages your architectural triumph. It's hard for a twin to stay on track and complete things, and this could contribute to the higher incidence of attention deficit disorder among twins and more (see Appendix, page 363).

Separate activities and outings are a good idea all round. They will help you relate to each child and give them each individual attention without the other twin getting in on the act. At 14 months or so, after a short separation of, say 20 minutes, your twins may greet each other with the kind of jubilation normally seen in long-lost Antarctic explorers who have just found their way back to base.

Many twins are never out of each other's sight, and this soon begins to tell. It can then be very traumatic if they have to endure a separation, if for instance just one of them goes to play at a friend's, or has a trip to hospital for emergency treatment.

When you organise separate outings, they needn't be ambitious. Even going down to the post-box or the corner shop in a borrowed single buggy can be exciting, while a picnic in the park or just the garden shed can be magical. If you have never had the pleasure of a singleton's company, it could be a welcome novelty for you too.

Any helpers or child-carers you have should make it easier for you to arrange individual outings, so explain that these are important. Otherwise grandparents and others may fail to see the point, especially if there's an older sibling who is, in her own way, very needy of time and attention.

As your children grow up, they're bound to ask lots of questions, most of them beginning with 'why'. 'Why am I a girl?' 'Why are those dogs doing that?' (Some queries are even harder to answer: 'Why is red?') Try not to address the same twin all the time (or first), even if one of them asks more questions or is more responsive to your replies. They both need explanations. It can be maddening, but be patient, and ready to repeat yourself if need be.

I feel so guilty that I don't give each of my twins as much attention as they'd like.

I've said that we parents of multiples have a special mission in life, but that doesn't mean having to be Super Mum or Super Dad. In fact you don't have to meet all your child's needs. Child development experts point out that if a child had no needs left, there'd be no incentive to learn new skills.

Fairness is another issue that causes parents a lot of angst. Yes, it's important to be as fair as you can, but life isn't fair. It's a tough lesson to learn, but it should be on the curriculum. As your children grow up, understanding life's inherent unfairness will help them deal with the inevitable ups and downs. In fact the great majority of parents seem to do very well, especially if you think of fairness in terms of a child's needs, not in terms of money. If you suspect that you are not even-handed, stop and analyse what you are doing and how you are spending your time. The chances are that you are doing a lot better than you imagine. If you're still worried, you can always talk this over with someone at Tamba Twinline (see Resources, page 372).

· *Individuality in the Wider World* ·

My three boys have very good comprehension and understand most of what is said to them and about them. I find the off-the-cuff comments and comparisons made about them at best ignorant and at times bordering on offensive.

As children get older, they spend more time with someone other than their mum. Many dads take a very active part in child-rearing, others less so. Mothers often worry about leaving Dad in charge of multiples because they think he won't be as aware of safety issues. Sometimes this feeling is totally unjust, and sometimes it isn't. Men don't always have the same attitude to hazards as women, so for peace of mind it can be worth talking this over. A few men can't even tell their young twins or triplets apart, something that needs urgent attention.

Whatever your children do away from you, whether it's at a school, at a friend's, or just out to the park with Dad, let each one share her experiences with you. Give each child time to talk, perhaps at bathtime or bedtime. Each needs to have his say in private sometimes, without the other child interrupting.

I'd want to know how Alex's day had been, and there was Kim, always jumping into the conversation to answer for him. Or vice versa. The only time it worked was if I put a video on to keep one child amused while I spoke with the other one. Sometimes I'd be so stressed from the effort of it all that I then couldn't remember who'd told me what.

Separate outings every so often are always helpful, perhaps even separate overnight stays at a grandparent's house. It's best to stay flexible on this point and let it evolve naturally. Forcible attempts to separate young twins for a day or more can backfire, as some mothers discover. If each child thinks of a weekend with Grandma as a punishment, because they didn't want to be separated, this does nobody a favour.

Different interests will evolve. Encourage these, without making artificial differences between your twins. One wants to do violin and the other one piano? Great. But maybe they both want to play the piano. Helping your children develop as individuals doesn't mean making them poles apart for the sake of it. It means helping each child choose what to do and who to be.

TODDLERS, OR THE TERRIBLE TWOS

I find that the toughest part of raising my two-year-old triplets is their constant desire for my attention. They do not want to share Mummy: 'My mummy's knee' – 'No, MY mummy's knee'. I had this image beforehand that I would have time with one whilst the other two played contentedly on the floor near us. Not so; they constantly interrupt each other, behave badly to get my attention for themselves and away from their brother, or sometimes I simply have three little boys clambering over me in an attempt to get in position for a story. Sitting on the floor with one on each leg and one between my legs sometimes works, for a very short time, until one boy grabs the book and runs off.

Toddlerhood is the time between one and three years, roughly between learning to walk and starting playgroup or nursery. It is a time of emerging independence, increasing negativity, unbounded curiosity and learning new skills (for you as well as your babies).

Typical toddler pastimes are finding out about the world, doing things for themselves and of course pushing Mum to the limit (just to establish what that is). What happens when you pull the cat's tail, climb the curtains or open that glass door with the suds behind it?

The main difference between having one toddler and having two or a whole gaggle is that your attention is divided, making it more difficult to keep them busy and out of trouble, especially when you are tired. Safety is a major issue and fighting is another, but along the way there is huge entertainment all round. Chapter 10, on behaviour and language, has more on fighting, while other toddler topics are covered here.

· *Safety* ·

As you are watching over or playing with one toddler, remember the other one (whoever said that there's safety in numbers wasn't a parent). Mothers of twins report a high incidence of injuries and accidents. A Tamba survey found that parents used more safety equipment with twins under five than when their older siblings were the same age. One particular danger is that rushing to the aid of one casualty can put the other twin at risk of injury.

Just as twins create more fun, they also make more mayhem. They egg each other on and they are physically capable of more: one small child cannot climb out of a play-pen, but she can if her brother lets her use his back as a step. Similarly, settees and bookcases may not withstand the onslaught from the power-pack that is two determined toddlers.

My two would use the banisters as a kind of game. Eloise climbed on the outside and Hilary on the inside, laughing and poking at each other between the bars until, inevitably, Eloise would either fall or be pushed off.

One toddler can jam the other one's fingers in a drawer and keep it painfully shut by leaning against it, or force the other's face down on to something as innocent as a piece of Duplo, necessitating a trip to hospital for stitches.

You are unlikely to get through toddlerhood totally without mishap, but you can reduce the risk of serious injuries by appreciating risks and anticipating accidents. Anyone – their father, grandparent, child-minder, baby-sitter, etc. – who looks after the children also needs to be aware of potential dangers. Cupboard catches and latches will stop or at least delay a toddler from getting at the contents, though they may not prevent one twin getting his hand trapped in the door by his brother or sister. Don't rely too much on catches: all chemicals should be well out of reach. Medicines too, of course. If some pills go missing, you may not even know which twin swallowed them.

A bolt high up on the inside of the front door will prevent your toddlers from running out into the street, but remove bolts and keys from bathroom and toilet doors, or fit a lock that only you can reach. On glass doors, use safety glass, safety film and perhaps stickers. Consider putting removable bars on upstairs windows, especially in the children's bedroom.

Kitchens, with their knives, flexes and cookers, hold obvious hazards. A strong stair-gate across the kitchen door helps keep your twins safe while you cook.

Heaters need fire-guards. Avoid wall heaters and electric or open fires altogether if you can. Irons are best kept well out of the way: even a cooling iron can burn. Make sure your domestic hot water supply is not boiling hot; turn the thermostat down if necessary.

Twins often enjoy bathing together at this age, but bathtime can be dangerous. Don't turn your back, even for two seconds, and never answer the phone or doorbell while they are in the bathroom. As a general guide, a child under the age of six is not safe on his own in the tub, and if unsupervised, even a seven-year-old can't be trusted in the bath with his twin. Friends with singletons may not believe it, but it's true.

For the sake of your nerves as much as anything else, put valuables and fragile belongings on a high shelf or in another room. It saves you having to say 'no' like a broken record.

I knew I had to hide all my favourite ornaments, like the china cats, but hadn't reckoned on the lamps. When I realised how fascinating my two found table lamps, I removed them from the sitting room for about three years in all.

Thinking ahead saves trouble. Keep your toddlers' finger-nails short. Avoid toys like hammer pegs: toddlers soon learn that you get better sound effects from whacking your twin's head than the pegs. Toys with string or rope can also be dangerous: one child may tie it around his brother's neck (or other parts of the male anatomy) and pull for all he's worth. If there's an older sibling, keep an eye out for his toys. Apart from the fact that the twins could upset him by destroying them, a big kid's toys can be lethal in younger hands.

Start keeping cot sides down from about 18 months, so that when the children begin to climb out they will have less far to fall. It is sometimes during holidays that they develop in leaps and bounds. For obvious reasons, avoid bunk-beds until they are much older.

While you are keeping one toddler out of trouble, the other one can quietly wander off and get up to something else. I don't mean to terrify you, but do think ahead. It's a dangerous world with more than one toddler. What's more, there is no such thing as a child-proof room: with twins, even a padded cell could be dangerous, as well as boring. Unless your toddlers are exceptionally placid, it is best not to let them out of your sight at this age. Supervise them, if only from a distance, while they explore. You won't be giving them much individual attention, but you can't do it all, and safety has to come first.

· *Clothes and Dressing* ·

For items such as underwear it won't matter, but on the whole your toddlers will prefer to have their own clothes, especially if you have a girl-boy pair. Dressing them differently, as suggested in the previous chapter, helps them develop as individuals, and children soon enjoy dressing and choosing their own clothes. It is also an important aid to safety. Toddlers should at the very least wear different outdoor clothes and wellingtons. A child who ventures out on to a busy road may well ignore an adult who calls him back by the wrong name, not because he is obstinate (though he may be) but because it isn't him that's being called.

It is one thing to get toddlers' clothes out and quite another to get them on their squirming bodies. The worst 10 minutes (or maybe hour) of your day is likely to be getting them ready in the morning. When they are very young, you have to dress them yourself, but it is not easy running after two or more toddlers who inevitably have so much more energy than you. Try to make dressing fun to encourage their co-operation:

- keep clothing simple (choose pull-up trousers and shoes with Velcro closures)
- be organised (getting clothes out the night before is a help)
- distract them while you dress them
- instead of rushing after them, try to get them to come to you.

It is faster to keep dressing them yourself, just as it is to continue spoon-feeding them, but sometime after their second birthday your children will need to learn how to do it. Some mums, especially if they have to get out of the house on time for work or to take an older child to school, find this stage absolutely maddening with twins, both of whom are determined to dress themselves, despite their complete incompetence. You just have to let them learn when they are ready, if necessary getting up earlier in the morning to do so. This stage lasts a long time with some children, but it passes, and you will benefit in the end.

· *Fair but Different* ·

Life is not fair, but this is a hard lesson to learn, especially when you're two years old. At this age, expectations of fairness are sky-high. If one twin gets a present or treat, or receives something which is in some way 'better', the other twin can feel punished.

Once parents realise the extent of their children's competitive spirit, they try very hard to be fair. But inevitably there will be occasions when they are treated unequally, for instance parties, Cub Scouts, etc. In the longer run, it may be preferable for children not to be treated fairly, but this is very difficult to do and at this age it is better to be even-handed.

Generally, the younger the children, the better it is for them to have presents which are roughly similar in concept or size, but presents needn't be identical. Although identical gifts are often acceptable, they can disappoint: if twins always receive the same presents, once one child has opened his, the surprise is spoilt for his twin. (To some extent you can get round this by sitting the children back to back when they unwrap presents.)

For substantial things, like a tricycle, the obvious choice is the same but in different colours. Ownership is important to youngsters, but some toys, such as a Wendy house, can be shared between them. When they get one present between them – it should be the exception, not the rule – you could also give them a tiny additional token gift each.

People can be amazingly unthinking, and as a parent, you need to encourage everyone to give your twins or triplets individual presents. Birthday cards which read 'Happy Birthday, Twins' should also be banned. People buy them because they exist, as do a lot of other stupid greetings cards.

Fair is not the same as equal; if you have one child with special needs, you know that already. It is better to give a child something she wants or that is appropriate for her.

Adults sometimes think they must spend the same on each child. One aunt was convinced it was only fair to pay a certain amount for gifts for her twin nieces, aged four. One Christmas this entailed her giving two presents wrapped up together to Sarah and only one, albeit larger and more valuable, to Frances. Neither girl could understand this, though. Frances was very upset, while Sarah gloated.

There will be times when you have to assume that they both want roughly the same thing. For example, if one child asks for a snack or a drink, it is sensible to offer one to his twin too, if only to save you getting up two minutes later.

Should you buy both twins clothes or shoes at the same time? You could spend a lot more if you do, so it is better to buy only for the one who actually needs new clothes. The other one may feel left out, but in time he will learn to accept it as normal. An ice-cream for the one who has not got a new winter coat is unnecessary and may make things worse. If hand-me-downs are available, try to alternate who gets new and who gets second-hand – not so easy with a boy-girl pair, though.

Like spouses, parents sometimes buy presents when they feel guilty. On the whole, it is better to be fair with time and attention than with money. Even this can be hard, though. Within a mixed-sex pair, for instance, the girl may have a longer attention span so you may read to her more. Differences are more obvious when one child has special needs.

· *Tantrums* ·

You may think that being flawlessly fair will guarantee peace. But toddlers don't work like that. The bad news is that tantrums are an inevitable part of growing up and most toddlers have at least one a week. They happen most when a child knows just what he wants but can't understand why he won't get it there and then. The good news is that they're not your fault, whatever onlookers seem to think, so you don't have to worry that you're failing as a parent.

Children do grow out of tantrums, but twins – especially boys – can go on having them longer. You may find that one of your toddlers flies off the handle more readily than the other, or that they set each other off.

I found that only Paul would start tantruming, but if I got overheated in the process, David would go bananas too, perhaps from fear.

You can help prevent tantrums by:

- being consistent but firm
- giving your toddlers plenty of attention
- giving way on unimportant issues (good practice for the teen years, too)
- avoiding unnecessary temptations, such as the super-market check-out with all the chocolates
- setting a good example: chances are that you often raise your voice, if only to make yourself heard above the twin din, but it pays to keep the volume and the emotional temperature down.

During a tantrum, shouting or smacking usually prolongs the agony for all concerned. A hug can help calm a child, but he may just need to be left, as long as you keep an eye on him to make sure he's safe. Turning your back on him to busy yourself with something else is ideal. But don't forget his twin: he may take the opportunity to wander off and cause his own brand of havoc while you are dealing with his brother's outburst.

After the storm, carry on as if it hadn't happened. It shouldn't alter anything. If you weren't going to buy him a sweetie, don't get him one now. This is hard, especially if your toddlers have chosen to tantrum in unison in the supermarket, but they have to learn that blowing an emotional fuse is completely pointless. (See Chapter 10 for more on bad behaviour.)

· *Potty-training* ·

Many mums dread this stage, but potty-training two or more toddlers isn't usually as difficult as they expect. It can however be messy, as it's hard to keep an eye on both at once. That is, assuming your twins are ready to come out of nappies simultaneously. They may not be. Even with identicals, there can be an interval of months between them. Children also vary in the order they develop: some have bladder control before bowel control, and vice versa.

> *They were both ready together when they were two and a half. Once they both did poos just as they'd got up from their potties and they both trod it into the carpet. Weeing was less of a problem, though both girls usually managed to store at least one settee's worth of wee in their bladders, to be released as soon as my back was turned.*

If you've done it before, you know that you can afford to be relaxed and take the long view. Don't rush anything to do with potty-training. Forcing the issue is counter-productive. And you can ignore bragging mothers, including yours if she claims you were clean by nine months (Gladstone was said to be, but politicians have been known to lie). Until the age of two, a baby's nervous system hasn't developed enough to control the muscles involved. There is all the difference in the world between 'catching' poos in a potty and real toilet-training, which demands both understanding and control.

Watch for signs that one of your toddlers is ready: she

may for instance start tugging at her nappy when it is wet or dirty.

If possible, start potty-training in warm weather soon after the children's second birthday. There are two main methods, but either way you need enough potties and eternal vigilance. Keep their clothing simple and easy to remove, or leave their bottoms bare altogether.

Either sit your children on their potties for a few minutes at a time, however long the toddler is happy with. At this stage, youngsters know what toilets and potties are for, so just wait till they either produce something or get bored. Bowels often move about 20 minutes after breakfast, so this is a good time. Congratulate the one who produces a result, but don't go overboard in your praise. If you show too much appreciation your child may offer you 'gifts' of his stools!

Alternatively, take off your toddlers' nappies for an hour or two to begin with, then for longer and longer. Keep the potties handy but don't make either child sit on one unless you see him leaping about, holding his crotch, wriggling or crouching down quietly in a corner (where the potty isn't). You will inevitably have accidents, but one day success will come.

Don't worry if only one toddler gets the idea. Twins are great imitators, so be patient and you may find that the second child is potty-trained for you. One note of caution: watch out for the toddler who empties his potty triumphantly over his twin's head.

You will soon reach the stage where you take potties with you when you go out. Terry pants are useful for outings, as are old towels in the seat of the buggy. You can usually rinse the buggy later with a garden hose.

Of course, toddlers still need nappies at night for a while, perhaps till the age of three or more. Throughout childhood, plastic mattress covers save time and effort, not just for poo and wee, but for the odd vomit or nosebleed too.

· *Playing* ·

Playing is what toddlers do instinctively. Actually all children play from an early age. Those first interactions a baby has with his mum, with eye contact, murmuring and stroking are all forms of play. As youngsters become mobile, and their horizons expand, their playthings become more sophisticated.

It is sheer joy to watch twin toddlers at play together. However, things can change quickly. One moment your little darlings are entertaining themselves beautifully, and the next minute one of them decides to use a toy as a weapon against his playmate. For this reason, many playthings suitable for your children's age can be hazardous with two or more. You also need to supervise your toddlers more closely.

Unless they are very robust, toys get broken more easily with multiples, causing disappointment all round.

Multiples make more mess, and you may decide to abandon experiments such as finger-painting. However, you could let them paint outside, or on a plastic tablecloth on the floor. One mother of two budding graffiti artists allowed them to draw on one designated wall outside the downstairs toilet. 'This worked very well,' she reported, 'though they did bicker over how much wall they should each have, until I painted a vertical line down the middle.'

A rocking horse can squash little fingers. Outdoors, a swing can be downright dangerous. The seat of the moving swing can hit the other twin on the head and knock her unconscious. You might think a see-saw would be brilliant for twins, but it too can cause injuries and thus rarely works out well. If you are considering outdoor toys, you are better off with a slide, trampoline, Wendy house or, best of all, a sandpit. This will exercise their imaginations yet consume hardly any of your energy.

When toddlers co-operate, it is heaven. Imaginative play tends to work really well with twins or more: plenty of customers when playing restaurants, lots of patients when playing hospitals.

When they're in less co-operative mode, playing or reading with them is enjoyable all round and also prevents arguments. But it is hard, to say the least, to play with one and not the other. One twin will be magnetically attracted to whatever the other one is doing and your attention will once more be divided. Obviously, the presence of a sensible older child or another adult is helpful, but most of us have to manage on our own as best we can.

One problem is fighting over toys. When twins fight they tend to do it with the gloves off, without much awareness of the damage they inflict. Who owns what, anyway? Some toys may be 'sharing' ones, but what about the Duplo and other bricks? If each has his own, they either play separately, or co-operate and get the bricks mixed up – and then squabble.

When they do fight, I take that toy away and offer them something else, or preferably a choice of several toys, to interest them. At this age, memories are mercifully short!

It is good for each child to have her own toys, although you'll naturally want to avoid unnecessary (read expensive) duplication. Possession is a basic human instinct, while taking turns is not. There's no evolutionary advantage in sharing or being kind, so children need to learn to do this. A youngster with her own playthings and her own box or shelf to store them:

- may be more careful with them
- may learn (eventually) to put them away
- may fight less.

· *Getting Out and About* ·

You will still use a buggy for most outings. A couple of toys in a bag are useful to keep your toddlers amused. Or take a small selection of reading matter: toddlers devour books, literally.

It is tempting to keep twins in their buggy till the age of four or so, but they need to walk. The trouble is they can choose different directions. Personally I would let them use their feet when possible, but take the buggy along in case they get fractious or fed up.

Reins that double as pushchair harnesses give you flexibility. Leather reins tend to work better than fabric. Reins also give your children freedom, though they can get tangled up (more so, inevitably, with triplets).

A buggy does reduce the chance to explore, but it doesn't seem to have much impact on road awareness. In practice, a child under five can't cross the road safely and he may be unreliable for years longer. Genuine traffic awareness is pretty rudimentary until the age of ten or so – shocking but true.

On car journeys, singing or listening to cassettes helps keep toddlers content enough for you to concentrate on the road ahead. According to research, nursery rhymes may even be a valuable aid to language development – if you can stand the repetition.

In the car, the main trouble with multiples at this stage is likely to be screaming, shouting or scratching each other, any of which can distract you. If this happens, just pull in and get them to stop.

I was against smacking but had no qualms about giving a sharp tap if they were acting up. Screaming and howling while we're on the motorway is definitely too dangerous to allow.

Another potential difficulty is the buckle on the child seat. It depends a bit on the model of the seat, but some youngsters soon discover that they can undo the buckle. Again, this practice is something you need to stop as it can be so dangerous.

Getting toddlers into and out of the car can be a pain if you have to do it more than a couple of times a day, and sometimes they nod off in the car seat just when you need to get out. If you are picking up an older child from school, you could ask another parent to bring her out to your car for you when this happens.

· *Leisure* ·

Yes, you will get to go out and enjoy yourselves, though some outings are more of an effort than they might be with only one toddler in tow. Even going to the park is demanding when twins decide to career off in different directions. An enclosed children's play area is obviously easier, although it still leaves you with the job of pushing two swings at the same time.

Dress your children simply for such outings, with wellingtons if wet, so that you don't mind if they get messy. After all, part of the fun of a rainy day is stamping about in puddles.

For safety's sake, it is inadvisable to go swimming with children this young unless another adult comes along to help in the water, as well as the changing room. Formal swimming lessons may also be out of the question, since some instructors insist on one adult per child. It may be better to wait till your children are a bit older, then enrol them in a class where a parent is not needed in the water. Don't worry if this means your children cannot swim until the age of six or seven. It's a social issue, not a safety one: a young child who can hold his own in a warm calm pool is no safer than a non-swimmer if he falls into an icy canal or a choppy sea.

Theme parks and funfairs are hard going without adult help. Many mothers find outings like these so demanding that they are simply not worth the effort (or the expense). You may feel that your children don't get many treats, but all these things get easier as they get older, when they are also more able to appreciate them. Besides, fun though they may be, theme parks are not one of life's essentials. A varied and stimulating home environment, with plenty of adult attention and opportunities to make friends, is good enough. Make the most of the outings you do go on: talk to each of your toddlers in turn about what you've seen and done, and be sure to make eye contact with each.

· *Going Visiting* ·

The other element to triplet motherhood that has made me very resentful is that everyone visits me. Friends with singletons assume that it is OK to visit but not to return the invitation. Neighbours with a new infant invited themselves to our home to show off their baby to the boys. We are constantly excluded from family meals and occasions.

Dropping in on friends can be exhausting if multiples overwhelm the host, especially those with only one toddler. If they start breaking things, it can also be embarrassing, and there could be tears all round. But don't give up. You can make it easier on yourself.

- Ask your friend to hide away the most fragile objects or most prized possessions. Perhaps her child could agree beforehand on what toys (if any!) he is willing to share with your tribe.

- Break up the visit with a meal, a picnic or just a walk in the park. Being outdoors helps burn off energy.
- Meet somewhere neutral: the park or a soft-play area at the leisure centre, for instance.
- Attempt short visits rather than day-long marathons.
- Use these gatherings strictly for the children's benefit and give up on meaningful conversations with your friend. You can always catch up on the phone some other time.
- Visit at times such as weekends, when you or your friend may have another adult around to keep an eye on the children.
- Take only one of your toddlers with you if possible. Better still, organise a morning's exchange with another parent of twins of a similar age, so that you have one of her children and she has one of yours. Many mothers find this an ideal solution as it helps when visiting and encourages their children to develop as individuals.

· *Having Friends Round* ·

Thanks to sheer numbers, your children can dominate the situation. Twins may even spend the afternoon sparring over the right to play with the visiting child, with the result that she toddles off to amuse herself on her own.

Occasionally, your children may gang up against the guest, despite the fact that they were all best mates the previous day at toddler group. A rough and unequal struggle can result.

Speaking to other parents of twins shows that, unfortunately, this is not unusual. Some add that having friends over to play was a problem that persisted well into their twins' schooldays. Here, parents of triplets can be at a distinct advantage. One mother says that her problems were invariably over if she invited one child in to play with her three girls.

If you have twins:

- Invite two children over to play.
- Try swapping one child for a couple of hours with another parent with twins.
- Have one little friend round while one of your toddlers goes to a grandparent, aunt, or to visit another friend.
- Play a game with one of your children while the other one plays with the visitor (not easy, but it can work).

You may find you have to give up having friends over for a while, until your children can cope with their jealousy and competition. If so, try not to worry, but do make efforts for them to have separate solo outings, so that each twin has individual opportunities.

· *Birthday Parties* ·

At last, one area where twins or triplets really mean economies of scale! In the early years, one party for both (or all) is plenty. Besides, friends and relatives are shared at this age. Even later on, sharing a birthday tends not to be a big issue for the kids.

However, they shouldn't have to share presents or cards, so discourage people from giving these jointly. If each twin has suggested his own guest-list, you could ask each guest to bring a present just for the child who invited him (this works only if each twin invites the same number of friends).

Nor should children have to blow out the same candles on one cake. You could have two cakes, or two sets of candles on the cake. This works well for several years if you have a cake in the shape of a log, say, or a train (until there are too many candles). Most parents of multiples sing 'Happy Birthday' as many times as they have children.

Watch out for games which only one person can win, such as musical chairs. One of your toddlers could be elated from his win, while his twin is either in the slough of despond or throwing a tantrum (not unusual at birthday parties anyway, even with singletons). You can try playing pass-the-parcel with two parcels, or opt for less competitive games. Avoid situations where one or more children who are 'out' can rampage around the house getting into mischief. Here another adult is a great help.

· *If You Have a Difficult Day* ·

Toddlers not only get into everything but seem to do it all on much less sleep than they needed as babies. The loss of one or both daytime naps is something a parent has to get used to. You can, for a while anyway, encourage them to nod off by wheeling them around the streets in their buggy at strategic times of the day, or going for a drive. If your toddlers do sleep in the day, use this time for yourself, not for chores. If only one dozes at a time, make the most of it by spending a few uninterrupted moments with the other child. He will benefit and so will you. Many a wild child becomes delightfully manageable on his own.

How else can you cope with all that exuberance, especially when your own get-up-and-go has got up and gone?

1   Minimise chores. Give up all non-essential housework and enlist your children's help with some of the others. Toddlers can enjoy 'polishing' the banisters while you vacuum. Admittedly, everything takes longer with that kind of hired help, but you will at least get something done.

2   Try to get through one day at a time without conflict, even when you have to repeat yourself like a tape loop

to keep your toddlers out of trouble. It is less inflammatory to tell them off by calling their behaviour 'silly' rather than calling them 'stupid'.

3   Mess creates stress, so keep things reasonably tidy. The more toys there are out, the less kids play with them, so keep some things hidden away. But there is no need to be obsessively tidy.

4   Have one or two activities or big toys that use up energy, for instance trampolining or bouncing on an old mattress on the floor. Or just get a few giant cardboard boxes to play around with (but watch out for any sharp staples).

5   Go out at least once a day. Toddler groups and one o'clock clubs are good ways for them to burn off excess energy, while you get to sit down.

6   Use different rooms for a change. Your toddlers could scribble at the kitchen table for a while, then play with bricks in the bedroom, before blowing bubbles out in the garden or the bathroom. You can picnic in your garden, or even under the kitchen table if it's raining.

7   Use television wisely. There are some excellent programmes for the very young. However, sitting glued to the set for too long can make children unbearably overactive later.

8   When they get restless, you can put on some music and dance together. A few crisps and a couple of drinks make an impromptu party.

9   Try not to let your children get overtired. If they are whiny and worn out but won't nap, sit and read to them together. Enjoying books quietly doesn't take much energy on anyone's part and helps develop language skills.

10 Nobody can go straight to sleep when they've been jumping about just before bedtime. Twins especially tend to overexcite each other, so help your toddlers unwind with a predictable and calming evening routine.

Chapter Nine

RELATIONSHIPS

We wish the world would realise that having three children at once does not mean that your ability to love them is divided by three. They mean as much to us individually as any singleton means to his parents.

All the same, sheer logic suggests that the fact of being born a twin or triplet will affect almost every relationship, and so it does, if only because there is someone else who is exactly the same age, making the same demands on parents. Also, the number of children in the home makes the number of possible relationships within the family that much greater.

Twins are not the same as one child, nor are they just two children very close in age (so-called Irish twins, though in Ireland they are known as American twins). They are exactly the same age: obvious maybe, but it is the crux of the problem. How does one deal with bedtime stories? Whoever goes first leaves the other trailing in second place.

There'd be terrible trouble over who got kissed goodnight first. At two and a half, both boys would lie in bed calling out, 'My arms are open.' I had to have a mental rota.

Twins may need the same things at the same time, but they can't usually have them, so they must learn to take turns, which some twins do sooner than singletons. In the process, there can be fierce rivalry.

· *Within the Twinship* ·

Twins usually spend more time together than they do with anyone else (including their mother), which is bound to be an important factor in the closeness and intensity of their relationship. Love–hate is a good description for many twin relationships; good–bad is another. There are many positive aspects of twin relationships, such as:

- affection
- mutual support
- co-operation and encouragement
- stimulation
- sympathy
- empathy and understanding.

There are also less attractive aspects, like:

- dominance or dependence
- competition
- collusion
- exclusivity.

It is, however, a bit simplistic to define characteristics in terms of good versus bad. Both positive and negative features may just be different ends of the same spectrum. When support and co-operation become extreme, for instance, or surface in less acceptable ways, the result may be little short of aiding and abetting.

I doubt if at the age of three Oliver could have got the bucket stuck around his chest, but with Anthony's assistance he managed it. However, neither of them could get it off again. He was stuck, with the handle round the front and the pail part of the bucket sticking out of his back. Both were giggling helplessly. And so was I. But my laughter turned to panic when I realised

I couldn't remove the bucket in time to fetch his older brother from school.

Competition

Rivalry can be a good thing. Many parents comment that competition brings out the best in their twins, whether on the sports field or in the classroom. Your twins may even try to outdo each other by helping with household chores – if you are lucky.

> *They'd both be champing at the bit, wanting to wash up or set the table, but as soon as one started helping me and showed he was enjoying it, the other would give up completely, find something else to do and simply fade into the background.*

An element of competition and even conflict is normal. According to some psychiatrists and psychologists, trying to eliminate competition altogether could cause fresh problems within a family.

Of course, it can be unhealthy and lead to fighting, a topic covered in Chapter 10, which deals with behaviour and language. In any contest, only one twin can win. This tends to accentuate any differences between them, with one taking up the leading role and the other following.

Some parents mind this very much, believing that their twins should be strictly equal, while others are happy to acknowledge it openly in front of their children. 'His brother's the dominant one,' a mother may say without inhibition, even though hearing this could have an effect on the dependent twin's self-esteem and may stop him from ever trying to take the lead. Parents can't shift the balance of power within the twinship, and perhaps they shouldn't try, but they can promote each child's individuality and sense of worth. This topic is covered in Chapter 7.

Comparison

Twins may enjoy being compared; after all, this is one way in which they can assert their personalities. Comparisons can become invidious, however. One of the children may become the 'bad' one on a long-term basis and become a scapegoat for everything that goes wrong. Sometimes parents or grandparents encourage this in subtle ways, either by saying, 'It's always Katy' or by just failing to express surprise when one particular twin misbehaves.

Obviously, nobody is ever wholly good or wholly bad and the assumption would be unfair. It gives neither child a chance. It's hard for the supposedly 'good' twin, who may have trouble living up to her halo, as well as for her sibling.

Scapegoating does of course happen in families without twins, but it is more awkward to handle when it involves children of the same age. One occasionally sees the reverse of this phenomenon, with one twin taking the rap for his twin's misbehaviour.

Understanding

Many, perhaps most, people assume that twins have some sort of tacit understanding and are able to share their feelings without verbal communication. Some twins seem to think so too. 'I don't need her to tell me anything when she's upset,' remarks one woman about her twin. 'I always know what's on Iris's mind.' 'Ask me – I always know what Oliver thinks,' says one seven-year-old boy.

A minimum of communication sometimes seems enough. For example, one mother took her one-year-old twin boys out shopping:

I was in a bookshop with Alex and Kim facing each other in their pram. Alex made a few noises, Kim gurgled fluently in reply as if telling a joke, and they were off in fits of giggles.

It brought business in the shop to a standstill as people gawped.

Same-sex twins versus boy-girl pairs

It is often agreed that identical twins tend to be the closest and most supportive of each other, even if they are some-times bitter rivals. Boy twins have earned themselves something of a reputation for being a handful. Girl twins tend to be more biddable but can also be trouble. Girl twins, especially if identical and dressed in attractive matching outfits, often receive a great deal of admiration, and like supermodels some expect to be the centre of attention.

Non-identical twins can also be very close, and some pairs are also very alike physically. boy-girl pairs are perhaps the least similar, to look at anyway. Among twins, their relation-ship tends to be the least exclusive, but it can still be very supportive. Often the girl is more advanced socially and physically and may take on the role of protector or 'mother' to her twin, something her brother may either enjoy or resent, especially if she bosses him about. The tables may turn in the teen years; this is discussed in later chapters.

The behaviour of boy-girl twins is often less stereotypical than it might have been had they been brother and sister born as singletons. The boy, for instance, may be quieter and less aggressive, much to his parents' relief.

Triplets

Three is an unstable number: many mothers reckon quads would have been less trouble. Although there are exceptions, triplets in many families don't always all play well together. One is often left out. This may either work on a sort of rota basis or with the same one of the three always being excluded, a situation which is hard to handle. An identical pair may cold-shoulder the third, non-identical member of their trio. Sometimes it is the one of different gender who is the odd one out; eventually he or she may come to detest being a triplet. This is obviously a tricky situation. All a parent can do is try to help each of the three develop as individuals and perhaps play down the significance of their triplet status.

Often, however, triplets club together to form a strong force:

My three musketeers (as I sometimes thought of them) were totally solid together when they were small. If ever one was in any kind of trouble, the other two would rush to the rescue. This gave me great satisfaction, but occasionally it led to problems. Once one of them broke a window. I never found out which. Their solidarity was worthy of the most militant trades union.

· *In the Womb* ·

'They start as they mean to go on' is the dire warning many midwives give pregnant women who have a very active baby. Don't worry – this is not necessarily true. Babies do however have some life before birth. So what kind of life is it?

As young babies, twins play together from the age of a few months old, far sooner than do most singletons. They may start interacting in the womb. Some experts now think that particular patterns of behaviour, or aspects of twin relation-ships, have their roots before birth. Alessandra Piontelli, an Italian psychoanalyst, has studied unborn twins with ultra-sound and concluded that they displayed some important characteristics before birth.

No two twins, even monozygotic, behave exactly the same in the womb. Some twins appear to seek out contact with the other twin, while others exhibit avoidant behaviour, shunning the touch of their twin. In some of the pairs Piontelli studied, these traits seemed to continue after the birth. The one cautionary note: Piontelli studied the children herself both before and after birth, and to date nobody has managed to replicate her results on a more objective basis.

There is, however, evidence that fetuses have some basic ability to learn before birth, and they have both short-term and long-term memory. It would be surprising to us modern parents if they didn't, although not so many years ago the months spent in the womb were thought of as a complete void, and babies were believed to think and feel nothing until the moment of birth.

· *Birth Order* ·

Being a twin is a race, and I won it.

Strangers often ask which twin is older: it's the most common question after 'Are they identical?' Before long, your children will be asking you too.

Unless you got them dreadfully shuffled in the ward and lost their plastic bracelets, at least you and your partner will know which twin was born first. But should you tell?

While some parents are open with this information, others like to keep it to themselves and may not even tell their twins, at least not for a long time. The truth will out eventually. In the UK, birth certificates include the times of birth for multiples; hospital records and your GP's notes will also record the birth order. However, some parents prefer to keep it a family secret for a while. You can probably get away with telling the children themselves that they were born at exactly the same time, for a while anyway.

The trouble is that once you have spilled the beans, the news is out for good – but does it matter?

Yes, it matters a lot, not to me but to my in-laws, who are Indian and regard the first-born boy as especially important. I hadn't realised it would be this way. If I had, I'd have kept it hushed up.

It also matters a lot in Jewish households. On the eve of Passover, the family Seder meal includes the recital of the Four Questions, traditionally by the youngest child. You might need to know which twin was the younger.

Rank is often important to an older sibling. Perhaps this is to be expected; after all, a big brother's status within the family depends crucially on the fact that he was born first. Once he knows the twins' birth order, he may accord the first-born much more seniority, or use it to explain different characteristics between the twins.

Often the first-born is indeed the dominant partner, though whether this is cause or effect is not certain. Research also suggests that the second-born twin often smiles more and is more eager to please. This applies especially to non-identicals of the same sex, but is by no means a universal rule.

Children can sometimes benefit from knowing their birth order. The shy, retiring twin may get a boost from learning that he was born first, ahead of his more assertive sibling.

Many twins like to know their birth order because it is the one thing they have which makes them different from each other. On the other hand, some regard it as unimportant. As one identical twin says:

My brother and I came from the same egg. We were conceived at the same time and it is just a question of chance as to who poked his head out first.

Being the elder can be a disadvantage. Some people expect the first-born to be taller or more intelligent. Do they seriously think a few minutes makes much difference? Katya was older than her non-identical sister by eight minutes, which also made her the eldest of a family of six children. She knew this from an early age and it was a huge responsibility because she was expected to behave better.

Whether and when you tell your twins is up to you. On the whole, it is probably best to tell them in childhood rather than wait till the teen years or later, but the decision is yours.

I could never bring myself to tell them, because every time my girls asked who was born first, they were always in the middle of a flaming row and wanted to know just so they could decide how to settle the argument! It seemed the wrong moment when they were so het up, so I didn't tell them until they were nearly 10.

The elder may not always be the one you think: in some parts of Africa, the second twin is considered older, in fact senior enough to have ordered his twin out first to ensure the world was ready for him!

Favouritism

You like Gareth more than me.

Having a favourite is very common, as mentioned in Chapter 4 (page 108). This is very natural and often sorts itself out. In time you may even find your preference reverses completely.

However, favouritism can persist and there may be lasting inequality in the feelings a parent has for their twins. If so, ask yourself why. Is it the first-born, or the boy of a boy-girl pair? Prejudice may do both your twins a disservice. However, it is widespread. There's ample data to show that parents who think of one twin as better in some way to the other one usually favour the twin who left hospital first. This bias can last for 20 years or even more.

Is your favourite child achieving more? This could be one effect as well as the cause of your feelings. If so, try to help the less able twin achieve his potential. He may be almost as able: parents often exaggerate minute differences and ignore the fact that twins are usually more similar to each other than to anyone else on earth.

What should you do if you have a favourite?

- First of all, don't feel guilty. This only makes things worse. As the family therapist Audrey Sandbank says, it is important not to get too hung up about favouritism.
- We all like some things more than others. Accept your current feelings as a fact of life, but avoid dwelling on them or making them too public, especially in front of the children.
- Do your best to avoid labelling and comparing. Labels change.
- Try to act fairly, however hard this is. Fair is not necessarily equal. A naughty child should not go unpunished, nor a good child unrewarded, just because he has a twin.
- Don't overcompensate. If you try to make it up to the less favoured one, you may reinforce unacceptable behaviour and make him even less favoured!
- It may not be you who has a favourite, but someone else, like your partner, a grandparent or a child-minder. It does happen. In this situation it is very important to be fair and get all the adults concerned to consider the points listed above; otherwise you could end up with alliances being forged. This can set the whole family at odds and also make discipline very tricky.

· *Relationships with Siblings* ·

Why can't I be a twin too?

It is hard being the brother or sister of a set of twins. Australian research suggests that 64 per cent of families with young twins have problems with the older child. This seems to apply especially when there are identical twins in the family, perhaps because there is too much emphasis (from the older child's point of view) on twin-ness.

Being between 18 months and three years of age when twins are born is particularly difficult, and no wonder. A toddler is old enough to appreciate what is going on, but too young to accept it. Imagine what it must be like to be upstaged by not one new arrival, but two.

Babies take up your time, energy and both your arms, all of which the older child still needs. The twins will probably sleep in your bedroom for months. Meanwhile logistics may mean that your toddler must move into a big bed now, or start walking because you cannot push his buggy as well as a twin pram. And all this around the time he starts potty-training or going to playgroup.

Whenever someone comes round, or stops to chat in the street, you can bet that all the attention is focused on the twins, with the older child being either ignored or asked how he likes being a big brother now. He may be expected suddenly to 'be big', but he doesn't know how and may not want to anyway. In fact it might be quite nice to be a baby too. Some children revert to bed-wetting or tantrums. Others – boys included – enjoy having a doll to be their twin for a while, or invent an imaginary twin.

A jealous older sibling may try a little attention-seeking or become aggressive towards the twins. This is very stressful to a parent already at the end of her tether; some researchers report a risk of child abuse in the siblings of twins.

Eventually it tends to sort itself out. Many older siblings become very mature and independent, as many only children do. But a few have lasting difficulties. Audrey Sandbank points out that siblings of twins need family therapy more often than twins themselves. By the way, the use of 'he' here is deliberate: compared with girls, boys find it harder to adapt to younger multiples in the family. Audrey Sandbank suggests this is because young girls can remain centre stage more easily. Her research also showed that the more children there are in a family, the better the older sibling manages. In later years your older child may get on famously with one of the twins, or else function happily on his own or relate to a younger singleton (if you are brave enough to have any more).

· *Helping the Older Sibling* ·

The earlier you start thinking about how your older child may feel, the more you can do to ease things for him.

Before the twins are born

- Don't tell him about the pregnancy too soon. Six or eight months is a long time to a toddler so you may as well wait till your bump shows, but do answer his questions. He won't like being left in the dark or having to piece together what is happening from overheard snippets of conversation.
- Avoid telling him the babies are just for him. They won't be much use as playmates for years to come. In fact, he may find them rather boring.
- Nor should you tell him he's getting twins because he's been so good. It is possible that there will be complications, for which he may then blame himself.

- Avoid moaning about your symptoms, even if you have a more troublesome pregnancy this time around. It could set him against the twins from an early stage.
- Make him feel special, but don't expect him to be too grown-up. He may find it daunting if you tell him you will need his help with the babies: he's far too young to act the parent! But you could explain that you will still want all his love and hugs (and vice versa).
- If there is plenty of time left and you were about to potty-train him, start him at playgroup or move him to a big bed, go ahead. It is best not to do these immediately before or after the twins are born.
- Try to find him a special older person to relate to, someone who will make a bit of a fuss of him. It could be an aunt, uncle, godparent, teenaged neighbour – anyone he likes who can be trusted to give him time and attention. These commodities will be in short supply when the babies arrive.
- If he has been going to a child-minder and likes her, consider letting this continue if you can, perhaps for a couple of hours every so often. The contact may help him.

When they arrive

- Someone your child likes (and you trust) is obviously the best person to look after him when you are in hospital.
- Let him come to the hospital to see the babies. Again, avoid moaning about your stitches, tiredness, cracked nipples, and so on.
- When you ring home, ask to speak to your son on the phone.
- Help your older child tell the new arrivals apart.
- Let him choose (even if it's with your money) something for the babies to have in their cots, maybe their first small soft toy. Tell him he can also decide who should get which.

- Encourage him to touch the babies if he wants to. Tell him 'Your little brother likes it when you do that.' Make sure little brother doesn't get injured. You may need to show a toddler how to be gentle with babies, just as if a tiny kitten had joined the household.
- Consider getting a special present for him.

When you get home

Many toddlers revel in this occasion, but sibling rivalry and regressive behaviour aren't always obvious right away.

> *I really thought Thomas was fine. He was interested in the twins, sweet-natured and acting perfectly normally, so I thought, 'no problem'. It wasn't until they were about six weeks old that he changed completely. He became very aggressive, wouldn't eat, wouldn't sleep and started wetting himself, which he carried on doing for nearly a year. I was at the end of my tether with three of them in nappies.*

Not every toddler reacts like this, but it is probably safe to assume that your older child's nose will be put slightly out of joint when the twins physically invade his home.

- Make time for him. If you have help, consider using it for the babies, so that you can devote yourself to your older child. Parents who have done this say it was the right thing to do and they would definitely adopt the same strategy again.
- Allow him to stay up later than the babies if possible. This may be hard on you at first, but he'll appreciate it.
- You may be exhausted, but try not to shout at your child.
- Give him plenty of cuddles and reassurance.
- Praise him whenever possible. He may be feeling negative at the moment, but you should try not to be!
- Some older siblings, whether boys or girls, are ready and

willing to assist with bathing, feeding, etc., but many are not and may resent feeling they have to. Give your older child the chance to get involved, but don't push him into it.

- Think about giving him a doll or teddy to change or feed while you look after the babies. He may lose interest after a while, but it can help. This is a poor time, however, for getting a family pet. Animals deserve more attention than dolls and soft toys and you really don't have time to settle one in.

- You are at your most vulnerable when feeding both babies at once, with no spare hands. This may be a good time to get out something special for him, perhaps a favourite video, a new jigsaw puzzle or just a cardboard box full of safe but interesting junk. You can make this a regular feeding-time ritual.

- When people turn up and coo at the babies or stop you in the street and peek into the pram, make a point of including your toddler. And if you are asked what the babies are called, introduce your older child first.

- Give your older child his own space and make sure his toys can go somewhere they won't be damaged by the all-chewing all-dribbling babies. This applies after they start crawling and going on the rampage too.

- Continue with his usual routine, such as bedtime stories, for as long as possible.

- Give him special outings on his own. He will have to get used to the new arrivals being part of the family, but all in due time.

- It could be a good time to start giving him weekly pocket money, but don't go overboard to compensate or give him a lot of sweets, crisps or things you might regret later.

- Don't leave him on his own with the twins. At this stage he may be less reliable than the family dog.

- If he is threatening to (or has already) hurt the babies, explain that he shouldn't, and try to give him an incentive to behave better in future. If he doesn't poke the babies' eyes all morning, he might be read a story, for instance. Reward systems can be very effective.

· *Siblings of Triplets or More* ·

The arrival of triplets or quads is particularly tough on an older child. Apart from the fact that you will be extra busy, triplets are unusual enough to hog all the attention. Again, make a point of introducing your older child – in his own right not as 'the triplets' brother' – and include him in any photos, whether they are for the family album or for publicity.

If you give any interviews to the press, make sure your older child gets a mention. In general, it is always a good idea to get the journalist's name and phone number in case you have any further thoughts before an article goes to press. You could even ask to see the piece to check it before it is published. Think carefully about what you say. An older child can be acutely embarrassed when personal details appear in the local paper. You may be, too. Remember, neighbours and friends may read what is published and you will have to live with it. Don't say anything you would mind seeing in print, for instance whether you had fertility treatment.

You may not get any fees for interviews and appearances, but it doesn't hurt to ask. Make sure you are not out of pocket: reimbursement of expenses is normal. Again, if it's not offered, ask. You could give your older child a small cut.

· *Parents and Their Feelings* ·

Becoming a parent makes you update your own view of yourself – certainly most other people see women differently once they are mothers – and lifestyle changes are far more dramatic when two or more babies arrive at once.

As a mum of twins, you will be busier and need to shift your attention quickly from one child to the other. The relationship between the twins themselves also affects how you relate to them: they may appear to need your approval less than a singleton might, for instance. Your feelings towards them could also be influenced by the presence of other people, be it your extended family arriving to help, or the au pair you drafted in. For all these reasons, mothers sometimes relate differently to twins.

> *I don't think I ever felt Alex and Kim really needed me, unlike my first son. The twins always seemed self-sufficient, and once they were about two or three years old they almost excluded me. I'd take them to the park and instead of being with them and pointing things out to them they'd toddle off happily together.*

The experience of another mother was entirely different.

> *Having twin daughters took me completely by surprise and I thought I'd never get used to it. I didn't want to breast-feed them, unlike my older daughter, whom I breast-fed for six months. But funnily I am much closer to the twins than to my first child. And they are more affectionate towards me. Perhaps it breaks all the rules, but there it is.*

Just as there is no such thing as a typical mother, there are no typical twins, so I can't make blanket generalisations about the relationships of mums and their twins. One important rule, though, is that the less happy you were to be pregnant with twins, the harder it can be to relate to them. That's one very good reason to sort out your emotions as much as you can before they arrive.

· *Parents as a Couple* ·

Gone are the days when a dad's job was over with the conception. In many families, fathers have a much more hands-on role. With twins, fathers often make an even more active contribution. Some dads find this is a time for role-reversal. There has been a sharp rise in the numbers of stay-at-home fathers, a route which might have been unthinkable a few years ago.

One of the pluses of having multiples is that it opens a new dimension for a father and gives him the chance of doing some applied parenting. When they are needed, the least promising men sometimes turn into the most adept fathers. Sadly, the opposite can happen too.

Multiples make a family special. Men often enjoy boasting about being the father of twins or triplets. In many ways, multiples can draw a family closer (like a war, you are all in it together). For some couples, though, twins are the last two nails in the marital coffin.

Parents argue most often about children and money, so there are plenty of opportunities there. The odds are stacked against those for whom the pregnancy was unplanned, who already have at least one child under the age of two, or who have triplets or more. Mothers often find that identical twins and twin boys (identical or not) impose particular strains on a marriage.

One father of twins, an architect, commented:

Le Corbusier said a house was a machine for living in. Well, if you asked me what a couple was for, for years I'd have said it was a machine for raising children. A very efficient machine, I might add, but that's all it did. After having twins there was nothing left in either my wife or myself for each other.

Twins tend to dominate a family, demanding most attention and dictating what can and can't be done. Dad and other siblings may be squeezed out of Mum's timetable by the constant demands of caring for multiples. A mother especially can wear herself out trying to be a perfect parent and home-maker (as it's called in the US). If you're tired and impoverished, it's harder to go out in the evenings: besides, could the teenager next door cope with baby-sitting two or three small children?

Horizons can soon shrink, isolating a family socially. Sex may become an unwelcome chore. If you can, take the long view of parenting. Children grow up eventually and you and your partner have to survive after the kids leave home.

There are no sure-fire ways of keeping romance or lust alive, or of ensuring you stay the course together, but the following can work.

- Go out together once in a while. It needn't be expensive if you join a baby-sitting circle. I know many mothers of twins who did not go out for two years or more after their children were born. When they finally did, some wondered just who this person was they had married. 'I recognised him, of course,' one of them joked. 'He was the bloke I used to meet at 3 a.m. traipsing the corridor with a crying baby while I was walking the other way with the other baby.'
- Join your local twins' club. Apart from some of the social activities you may be interested in taking part in, it may convince you that there is indeed life after twins – or triplets.
- Try not to argue over trivia. It is just not worth it. If you really feel like exploding over the dirty socks in the hall (again), why not just say, 'I really feel like exploding'?
- Every so often, have a candle-lit dinner. It can be in your own kitchen, but the point is that the atmosphere must be relaxing and make a contrast from the usual run of meals eaten on the hop.

- Pretend you've only just met your partner. This sounds daft and may not work for you, but many couples get a thrill from starting at the beginning with each other, flirting and thinking of intimate, sexy things to say.
- Try spending a whole evening (or however long you have) stroking each other everywhere but the genitals. Many people are driven to distraction by this arousal technique. Called sensate focusing, it is used in some kinds of sex therapy. If you want a non-scientific description, you could do worse than read David Lodge's 1991 novel *Paradise News*.
- Get some reliable contraception, ideally before you need it. Babies can be a form of birth control but, alas, they are not as reliable as the Pill, coil, diaphragm or . . . you get the picture. Women who have twins are often more fertile, and some have even had a second set of twins within a year or so. Even if you are not one of these favoured few, you don't want to lie awake at night worrying whether you are pregnant with triplets.

Chapter Ten

BEHAVIOUR AND LANGUAGE

We went for the day to my in-laws. Martha and David were two years old. In under three hours they'd stamped on the video, unplugged all the appliances, forcibly taken the aerial out of the telly, broken an antique clock and torn wallpaper off the wall. They ended the afternoon by squabbling under the dining table.

'Twins! How lovely!' This may be what a lot of people say, but these aren't exactly the words most likely to trip off your tongue when your twins act up. When they do, you will see why, in some African tribes, 'May you be the mother of twins' is considered a dire curse.

All children fight, don't they? Of course. But research shows that bad – or, to be PC about it, socially immature – behaviour is about twice as common in twins aged three than it is in singletons. Many parents discover that twins and triplets can be hard to control, sometimes to the point where they exhaust everyone around them. In a small number of cases, there is a connection between language and behaviour difficulties, which is why this chapter deals with both.

· *Bad Behaviour* ·

There is evidence that:

● temper tantrums in twins (see Chapter 8) may go on past

the stage when most singletons grow out of them
- twins can lack concentration
- bad behaviour can be common in school-age twins, especially identical boys.

None of this means that your twins will be a handful, and certainly not that they will be non-stop terrors.

> *My two boys were lovely at least 90 per cent of the time. It is just that in the other 10 per cent, when they went ballistic, I'd be at my wits' end. Often I couldn't guess in advance when it would be, though looking back – the boys are now 10 – I remember that they were most likely to act up when I was making an important phone call. They'd usually just shout, or else fight, and once Kim pushed Alex through a glass door.*

· *Why do Multiples Misbehave?* ·

Many factors can operate, so it's hard to target a single cause. Here are some of the possibilities:

- Multiples compete fiercely for mum-time. What surer way of getting attention?
- Twins often co-operate or collude. They egg each other on, are physically able to cause more trouble and may cover up for each other. Under these circumstances even experienced parents find it hard to keep the upper hand.
- While busy together, they may not listen. What does eventually get through (your shouting, for instance) can be very confrontational.
- Since they have each other, they may need less adult approval.
- Research shows that boy twins tend to have less contact with their mother and get less affection shown to them

than do two-year-old singletons. The reason's not known, but it might be significant.

- It is physically harder to restrain two or more children who misbehave, especially on outings.
- Some twins have delayed language development (dealt with later in this chapter), which is occasionally linked with difficult behaviour. It isn't always so, though; there are mischievous twins without any language problems at all. In fact, there can be a marked gap between how well they speak and read and how immature they sometimes act!
- If you are a single parent, it can be harder to stand firm on your own, though one obvious plus is that you don't have another adult disagreeing with your strategy.
- When one child has special needs, it is hard to know just how much discipline is right. In setting boundaries shouldn't one take into account his individual problems and not be too strict? On the other hand, the healthy twin also has needs and she may perceive her parents to be grossly unfair (there is more on this situation in Chapter 15).
- Research shows that some twins have attention deficit hyperactivity disorder (ADHD), which significantly affects concentration and learning. Having studied 2,300 families in Australia, Professor David Hay found that ADHD is almost twice as common in twins as in singletons and affects 16 per cent of boy twins and 8 per cent of girl twins. There's more on ADHD in the Appendix (page 363).

· *Pre-empting Problems* ·

Discipline is a hideous word, but all it means is acting appropriately within acceptable boundaries. It is an essential part of growing up and all children have to learn it. In a nutshell, these are the most important things you can do to get the best from your twins:

- aid their individual development (sometimes called 'individuation')
- give your attention fairly
- handle them consistently
- set a good example.

There are many different strategies and ideas which can help, depending on your circumstances.

- Try not to let them get bored or overtired, as they will be more difficult to handle.
- Be fair but firm. If you don't normally allow the kids to jump down from table without asking, don't make exceptions.
- Make sure you address each twin, using his name first. A child won't be in any rush to put on his shoes if he doesn't know who's being asked.
- Try to give the same amount of attention to each, if necessary using the kitchen timer to be – and be seen to be – scrupulously fair.
- Give each child a chance to have his say with you in private, for instance at bathtime or bedtime. Privacy is something multiples rarely get.
- Separate outings can be an eye-opener. If one of your little monsters becomes delightful on his own, then that, says twins expert Dr Elizabeth Bryan, is how he really is.
- Be positive rather than negative. It's better to hear 'Do go with Grandpa' rather than 'Don't be such a slowcoach.'
- A challenge or dare can help. An incredulous 'Can you really do up your shoes?' may work wonders, as can 'Bet you can't put the bricks away in two minutes.'
- Try to set boundaries – reasonable ones! When you have young children, it is pointless being obsessional about tidiness, say.
- Give simple reasons for your rules whenever you can.

Being rushed, mums of twins tend to make instructions short, but 'Just because' is maddening to children.

- Know when they are ill. Normally kids are naughtier far more often than they are unwell, but even parents who are doctors or nurses occasionally get caught out.

- If you are at the end of your tether or unwell yourself, don't be too ambitious. Scrap the trip to the supermarket if you can and just try to get through the day doing the minimum in a low-key way.

- Keep temptation away where possible. For instance, put cherished objects out of reach. And if you never put any coins in one of those Postman Pat rides at the shopping centre, your children won't act up on the occasions when you refuse to oblige.

- Stay in control yourself. Shouting unnecessarily just cranks up the aggression. It also makes you a poor role model.

- If you threaten your children, it has to be with something you would actually carry out. They will soon realise that you won't dump them on the dual carriageway if they scream in the car or get the neighbour's child in to finish their meals when they leave food on their plates.

- Try not to use food (or lack of it) as a punishment. It only makes meals more emotionally charged.

- Get help before a real crisis occurs. A friend who takes just one of the children for a couple of hours could defuse an explosive situation.

- If you have one, a responsible older child is a useful ally, but beware the big brother or sister who just likes bossing the little ones about.

- Always praise your children on the rare occasions when they admit to a misdemeanour. Owning up is a particular problem with young twins and they certainly won't do it if it results in punishment.

- Whatever has happened during the day, try not to put them

to bed on a bad note. Kissing and making up makes for sweeter dreams.

· *Coping with Double Trouble* ·

All the way home, they were hitting each other in the back of the car with the book I'd just borrowed from the library – it happened to be Toddler Taming . . .

Identical twin boys tend to mature most slowly and have earned a reputation for having the biggest behaviour problems. They need a really firm but no less loving hand. Many parents find that separate bedrooms for each boy help, but don't be too surprised if, having moved to a larger house to make this possible, they argue about the size of their respective rooms, and end up spending a lot of time in each other's bedrooms anyway . . .

Whatever your type of twins or triplets, they will inevitably have their trying moments. In time you will evolve your own personal style of dealing with these, but meanwhile the following advice will help:

- When your twins are naughty, express disapproval of what they did but assure them you still love them (e.g. 'I love you but I hate what you just did to your sister').
- Make the bad behaviour seem really boring. You may need to separate warring twins (more on this later), but giving the aggressor attention can reinforce bad behaviour.
- Don't smack, unless perhaps there is physical danger, such as when a child fiddles with the oven door or runs into the road.
- Get them to apologise whenever one has been tormenting the other(s). A churlishly mumbled 'Sorry' may be all you get. Well, you cannot expect miracles.

- Say sorry yourself when you get things wrong. It sets a good example. Besides, being fallible can excuse your mistakes in future . . .
- Try to avoid making one child a scapegoat, even if it is consistently one twin who misbehaves. When you are not sure who did a dirty deed, you can either let both off (which encourages collusion), or else punish both (OK, it's unfair, but a relatively mild and reversible punishment can work, and some parents find it also helps twins own up).
- 'Time out' in another room, or spent standing in the corner, has become a time-honoured method of discipline and usefully separates warring twins, but in the very young it only works when used for short periods of time, say five minutes for a five-year-old. The idea is not for the child to find something interesting to do (read: mischief), but to remove him from the scene of the crime. Of course there will be times when you want them to play separately for 45 minutes at a stretch, but it is best not used as a punishment.
- I don't think it is a good idea to send one twin up to his bedroom: he may end up disliking bedtime. Also, the one who is left playing downstairs may gloat – unfairly, if they've both been naughty.

· *Two Special Problems* ·

Should you stop them fighting?

Fighting passes eventually and young adult twins rarely come to blows, but it can seem an eternity until then. As one mother says:

> *The boys are nine and a half now and some days I still cannot go*
> *and have a bath in peace, or even use the loo, without World War*

*III breaking out. Last time, one tried to strangle the other with
his school tie.*

The cause is not often aggression in itself. School-age twins
– including the ones just mentioned – fight each other at
almost every opportunity, but never lay a finger on their
classmates.

The big question is whether or not to intervene. Parents of
singletons usually believe you should let them get on with it,
but you'd get a different answer from mums of twins who
have had to take one or other child to accident and emergency. Even then, hospital treatment may not deter twins
from getting just as physical in the future.

Methods that work with aggressive singletons are sometimes less effective with twins. One mother had trouble with
her three-year-old boys, one of whom had been hitting the
other on the head with a stick. When she removed the stick,
the offender cried bitterly and the victim was so moved that
he retrieved it and returned it to his brother, whereupon the
violence began anew!

One characteristic of fighting twins – or triplets – is that
when they fight they do so without any inhibitions or self-
restraint, causing far worse injuries than a singleton would
inflict on a friend or sibling. Perhaps serious fighting breaks
out because both are at a similarly immature stage of
development. Their lack of control may also relate to their
earliest days as babies, when they hardly knew where one
baby's body stopped and the other's began.

At one point, driven to distraction by frequent screams and
punch-ups, I asked each of my own boys, then aged eight,
whether they thought a grown-up should stop their fights.
Without hesitating, each said that I should. But they offered
no hints as to how best to achieve this . . .

Most parents of twins who have gone through these
phases advise playing things by ear. Let them get on with it

and sort themselves out if nobody is getting hurt, but make sure there are no potentially lethal weapons lying about. Your twins may well work it out of their systems within minutes and once again become the best of friends. But do keep an ear out for signs that things are getting too rough, so that you can intervene before they reach the stage of GBH.

Biting

> *The first two-word phrase one of my twins strung together was an indignant 'Bit me!'*

> *My girls were very pretty as toddlers, or would have been had they not given each other nasty bites on such a regular basis. This could be anywhere on the body, including their faces. As the teethmarks faded, they'd look like bruises, and I'm sure passers-by wondered what I'd been doing to them.*

One of the most frequent problems brought to both Tamba and MBF is that of biting two-year-olds. Audrey Sandbank and Dr Elizabeth Bryan warn parents that giving the perpetrator attention is often the last thing they ought to do. One mother, for example, resorted to carrying her two-year-old son constantly to prevent him biting the other two triplets. Of course, he got exactly what he wanted.

Biting tends to be within the twin or triplet group; they rarely bite outsiders. Often both twins bite each other, though in each incident there is usually a victim and perpetrator. A biting toddler is dangerous because she can do so much damage unchecked – and incidentally teeth carry bacteria.

The best method of dealing with an attack of biting is simply to remove the offender and give him minimal attention, to make the biting seem really boring and unrewarding. Whatever you do, don't let him see that his behaviour riles you.

Tamba's consultant family therapist Audrey Sandbank recommends picking up the victim and giving him two minutes of undivided attention. If the biter interrupts, explain that he has to wait because he was biting. He'll soon get the idea. The MBF's health visitor Rosie Ticciati makes similar suggestions, adding that you should first remove the biter to a corner and say firmly 'No biting.' Do be consistent and avoid raising your voice. Never mention the incident again as that too would be a form of attention.

Should you bite back? Some mothers advocate this, but it often makes things worse. If anything, it suggests to young-sters that violence in general and biting in particular are okay. It's a desperate measure and it doesn't work. There are Child Protection issues too.

· *Getting Help for Behaviour Problems* ·

There are several avenues of help for established problems, including:

- Tamba Twinline: you can discuss your difficulties with trained volunteers who are themselves parents of twins or more (see Resources, page 372). Tamba also has honorary consultants who may be able to help.
- Your GP or health visitor: they are unlikely to be experi-enced in dealing with multiples, but can still give useful advice and support and make appropriate referrals to other agencies. They can also get useful advice from the MBF, and either professionals or parents can make the first contact with the MBF (see Resources, page 372).
- Family guidance therapy: usually available locally (your GP can refer you). As Audrey Sandbank points out, this is an excellent method for twins and results can often be seen quite quickly. It works best when started

early, preferably before age five, but there are no firm rules on this. Warning: waiting lists can be long.
- An educational psychologist: especially if there are problems in school-age twins (discuss referral with your children's teacher). Difficulties at school need not be educational in nature for the child to qualify for being seen by an educational psychologist – they can be primarily behavioural or social problems.

· *Language* ·

Even back in the 1930s, it was known that the language of twins at ages two, three, four and five was subtly different from that of singletons. Since then, a great deal of research has confirmed this and has helped piece together a picture of language development in twins. There has been far less work done on triplets and more – most of this section is therefore about twins.

Language is a set of symbols for communicating thought, and can be written or spoken. Of course, children usually learn to speak before they read or write, so a child's acquisition of language generally refers to speech and how it is used. Language has many different components: making the right sounds (called phonology), using grammar (syntax) and conveying meaning (semantics). Acquiring language is a twofold process: understanding others, and producing speech.

How do children learn language? Although experts debate their relative importance, the main factors are:

- a child's innate readiness or ability
- intelligence, or understanding of the world
- imitation.

This last point is crucial. I will never forget the mother who brought her child to the hospital clinic because he hardly spoke. ''Course,' she added, 'he can say "Bugger off".'

With twins, the general trend is that:

- they are older than singletons when they say their first word
- each utterance is shorter
- sentence structure is simpler
- vocabulary is smaller
- baby-talk persists longer.

On average, twins are about six months behind singletons in language development. That doesn't mean all twins fall behind singletons. Many twins are very advanced in their use of language, and just because research highlights the ones who aren't, it doesn't imply your children will have problems.

Some of the factors that can delay language include:

- being male
- premature birth
- low birth-weight (whether premature or not)
- being in a large family
- being under-stimulated as an infant.

All these factors apply to singletons, too.

There has been and still is a lot of work in this whole area. One huge ongoing project is the Twins' Early Development Study (TEDS), which focuses on the early development of three common childhood problems – communication disorders, mild mental impairment and difficult behaviour. If your twins were born in England or Wales during 1994, 1995 or 1996 you may already have taken part in some of this study. TEDS has enrolled more than 15,000 pairs of twins, from families representative of the UK as a whole. The findings aren't just relevant to multiples. One result so far is that the same genes seem to play a part in problems with both language and general understanding.

· *Problems* ·

Does it matter if your twins' language is delayed? It is now becoming clear that language difficulties are often transient. In other words, they are a short-term delay, not a disorder. Findings from TEDS suggest that transient language delay is a separate entity from language disorder, and that it is mainly environmental in origin. In most twins, language delay has no long-term consequences for their education or their behaviour.

All the same, it is important for parents and teachers to be aware of possible language difficulties, because:

- there is sometimes a link between poor language development and bad behaviour, especially in twin boys (you might have guessed this, as behaviour is a way of communicating feelings)
- some twins with language problems early on will have trouble reading
- help can be given; it works best if started early
- good use of words is a key to success in other areas (even subjects like maths depend heavily on word power).

Reasons for language problems

The fact that a parent of twins cannot give each child undivided attention probably lies at the root of language delay, just as it does of many other difficulties in twins. Singletons from large families also tend to be less good with words, so perhaps the situation of twins is an extreme example of the same thing.

Researchers have found that there is one thing twins are very good at: responding quickly, though not necessarily to their mum. When the pressure is on, they obviously become expert at having their say.

Here are some of the reasons for language delay and problems in twins:

- With constant interruptions, parents of young twins are less able to have long conversations with their children.
- Mums of twins use simpler, shorter sentences. Obvious, perhaps, that with two toddlers you are more likely to cry urgently, 'Put that down!' than to explain patiently, 'Now, that's a very pretty vase I got as a present, and we don't want it broken.'
- Parents often talk to both twins at a time. In 'Paul-and-James come here' neither Paul nor James is an individual.
- Because of rivalry and lack of privacy, many of the conversations a parent has with each of her twins are really three-way events, so-called 'triadic communication', a confusing exchange like a dysfunctional telephone conference.
- When a mother speaks to one twin, her gestures and actions may, confusingly, have nothing to do with what she's saying. When you next feed your youngsters, for instance, you may well spoon food into one while carrying on an unrelated patter with the other baby.
- Mothers interact less with multiples – after all, it is easy to assume that they keep each other company.
- It is not quite clear why, but two-year-old boy twins may be spoken to less by their parents – and even seem to get fewer hugs than singletons. Many mums reckon they shout more at their boys, though.
- Twins often understand each other's needs and may use

body language, so it may be less important for them to speak to each other. This probably applies most to identical (MZ) twins.

- When twins talk, they often make the same mistakes, which reinforces errors and may even worsen them. Research shows that young twins aged two to four understand each other's speech well, even when it is full of mispronunciations. This doesn't happen with other children of the same age.

- Mothers may not bother to correct twins' inaccurate speech as much as they might a singleton's. It is partly pressure of time, but baby-talk can be attractive. As Audrey Sandbank points out, some mothers find it part of the undeniable 'cuteness' of young twins.

- Triplet language difficulties tend to be similar to those of twins, and they can be slightly worse. It all depends on how much individual attention the children get. But it is hard to generalise. Triplets with language disorders are a small group.

- Finally, prematurity, growth retardation in the womb, birth difficulties and genetic influences can all have a bearing on language problems. These can affect singletons too. The early environment is vital, as research confirms.

· *How to Encourage Language* · *Development*

Perhaps you cannot do much about prematurity or any medical complications your twins may have already had as newborns, but there are still plenty of ways you can help avoid language problems. There is no evidence that twins with language or speech delay have any difficulty with comprehension. This suggests that in most cases the potential is there. All you need to do is exploit it.

Some of the points below were highlighted by the La Trobe Twin Study in Australia. A few of the tips may be obvious to you, others less so. With twins, it's all about seizing opportunities.

- Starting from the tender age of four months, encouragement from parents can help language skills develop. Here is where time and attention, including the all-important eye contact, really matter. Spending time with the babies and talking to them individually is not only more fun than housework – it pays off. When speaking to them, make sure your actions match your words.
- When your twins start to speak, get them to say what they want. Life may be more peaceful if you continue to anticipate their needs, as when they were tiny, but this will not teach them to talk. If one baby just points at a cup and grunts, try saying 'You want milk?' In time, this helps him use words.
- One twin shouldn't talk for the other. Ask each child how playgroup was that morning. At first they may argue over who speaks first, but they will eventually take turns when answering questions.
- Ignore interruptions or attention-seeking behaviour. Setting an example yourself is good too, but easier said than done.
- Show them what good speech sounds like, without making a big thing of it by saying 'No, it is supposed to be . . .' Just repeat, in its correct form, the word your child has pronounced wrongly, ideally put into a simple sentence. The message will get through.
- If baby-talk persists, encourage them to realise that speaking better will help them get what they want more easily, make more friends and so on. This is tough, because many

grown-ups find lisping attractive. Your efforts at promoting good speech may be undermined by people who smile indulgently at your children's most immature sentences.

- Read to each child separately from an early age. If you can manage it, 10 uninterrupted minutes a day for each twin is far better than reading to both simultaneously for 20 minutes. The trouble is you need someone else – adult or older child – to keep the other twin entertained. Of course it is lovely to sit with a child tucked under each arm, so there is no reason why you shouldn't read to them together too if you want.

- An older child is useful as a role model, if he speaks well. It is often pointless to rely on a sibling who is only a bit older than the twins: apart from any rivalry, his speech too may be immature.

- Watch out too for the older sister or brother who dotes on the twins and gratifies all their needs. However handy this may be for you, it may not help the youngsters' development.

· *Language Development* ·

It is not always easy to know when there are real difficulties. Some language problems, such as a slight delay, vanish in time, while others need treatment.

An added complication is that normal children vary: they don't all learn to speak at the same age, though on the whole they do develop speech in a predetermined order.

In the first eight weeks of life, babies make basic noises like crying and straining. From two to six months, there is usually laughter, cooing and chuckling, often in response to what the mother does or says.

The stage between six and 12 months is sometimes called vocal play. Babies enjoy making sounds and begin to babble.

Twin babies usually babble to each other as well as alone. Towards the end of the first year words are finally produced – just single syllables to start with, and often the same sound for different things. A 12-month-old may say 'cak' to mean both 'cat' and 'nice', though obviously only in families that like animals. At this stage one may notice that babies with different mother tongues begin to make slightly different noises.

Between 18 months and two years, children form sentences which gradually increase in complexity. By the age of five, a child has already learnt much of his grammar.

Sounds are not all equally easy to produce. They tend to appear in this order:

Normally, by this age	*. . . these sounds are no problem:*
1½ years	p, b, m, h, w
2½ years	t, d, n, k, g, gn
3 years	y, f, s
4 years	sh, z, v
5 years	ch, j, l
7 years	th, r

There are differences from culture to culture. For instance, some sounds that are perfectly easy for, say, five-year-old Arabic speakers can still pose a huge challenge for English speakers at any age!

Spotting problems

The checklist below is a useful guide to spotting problems. You should suspect speech difficulties if one or both your twins shows any of these symptoms:

- is more than a year late mastering the sounds listed above

- uses mainly vowel sounds
- is hard to understand after two and a half years of age
- leaves out or substitutes consonants after the age of three
- distorts lots of consonants after the age of four
- talks with an odd rhythm or unusual pitch (e.g. monotonous, nasal, or too loud).

Other symptoms of language disorder include:

- not 'playing' with words by the age of one, or stopping babbling around then
- no response when spoken to at the age of one
- no spoken words (or fewer than six) by the age of one and a half
- no two-word phrases by age two
- unable to answer very simple questions by age two and a half
- no sentences by the age of three, or sentences which are only echoes of what the child hears
- baby-talk or very poor sentence structure after the age of four
- difficulty following a two-step instruction (like 'Go inside and take your jumper off') after the age of three.

If a child has trouble with sentence construction as well as with making sounds and interpreting meaning, there is likely to be a significant problem that needs treatment.

What you can do

The linguist David Crystal believes that by the age of seven or eight, the language delay of twins, often very obvious at the age of three, will have disappeared. This seems to be confirmed by others in the field – as long as the delay is fairly mild.

There are a few twins (and singletons) in whom language is so disordered that there are long-term effects on behaviour and education. An example is a pair of boys who were just about to start school when they were brought to the paediatric clinic, scarcely able to say a word. Obviously it's better to act before things get that critical.

The earlier parents take steps, the better. The outlook for both reading and behaviour also improves if any language problems are tackled by age four, and preferably by age three.

Although multiples can be prone to language problems, it's vital not to miss common causes. Learning to speak means imitating others, so normal hearing is essential. As a family doctor, I recommend a hearing test as a first step for any child (twin or singleton) who has any delay or difficulty speaking. Your health visitor or GP can arrange this. Hearing loss is more likely in children with recurrent ear infections, but every so often a youngster who has never had earache has a substantial hearing deficit.

Assuming that your children's hearing is normal and that nobody suspects a communication disorder like autism, what next?

If your twins are very young and the language problem is mild – say they are only a couple of months behind the expected stage in producing speech sounds – all they may need is individual attention. Reading to each separately on a daily basis, with his twin supervised in another room, is an excellent way of doing this.

Since about 5 per cent of children have some language delay and most children recover from it, there is some debate as to what else should or can be done. With anything more than the mildest delay, it is wise to get an assessment from a speech and language therapist. If possible, ask for a therapist who has experience of working with twins. Sometimes professionals aren't up to speed with multiples, or else they dismiss a parent's concerns with the catch-all explanation 'They're twins, they'll grow out of it.'

Your GP can refer you or you can access services yourself. You may have to wait some time for an appointment for an assessment, so don't delay setting the process in motion. While you are waiting, you can read to your children separately (if you don't already do this).

Identical twins tend to have similar language skills. All the same, it is not unknown for only one twin to need speech therapy, in which case one may gloat while the other is upset – and sometimes the one having therapy acts superior! This situation needs tactful handling. There are no easy answers, and you will need to:

- ensure that neither twin thinks he is now 'better' than his sibling
- help the twin being treated and reinforce what he's learning
- prevent his 'untreated' sibling from persuading him to revert to his old speech errors.

· *The Secret Language of Twins* ·

I have already mentioned that twins probably communicate from before birth, but how often do they use a private language that only they understand?

The secret language of twins (also known as idioglossia, cryptophasia or cryptoglossia) has been a subject of intense fascination for many years. True, a few twins do speak nothing but their 'own' language and every so often dramatic examples receive publicity.

Some researchers have suggested that in toddlerhood up to 40 per cent of twins speak a secret language that nobody else, not even their parents, can understand, and that the proportion may be even higher in identical twins. This sensational figure is probably an illusion, according to many experts. The private language can often be understood by outsiders who try hard. Research also shows that:

- young twins are good at understanding each other's speech and body language
- they make similar mistakes in speech
- because they tend to reinforce each other's mistakes, errors persist longer
- their language development can be delayed.

All in all, this is probably enough to give the impression that secret languages are common. If one listens carefully to a piece of so-called cryptoglossia, in many cases it's simply very immature speech, a kind of shorthand speech.

What if your twins really do share their own language? The answer is that it doesn't matter provided that normal language is also developing at the right time. Come to think of it, many of us, for instance husbands and wives, use our own private words. I'll spare you the examples as I'm sure you know what I mean, and we would be mortified if outsiders heard them. As long as we can and do speak normally with others, this is not important.

· *More than One Language* ·

Within our multicultural society, there are many families where youngsters speak one language with their parents and another with their grandparents, child-minder or at the nursery. Parents of children with speech delay often believe that the problem is due to learning more than one language at the same time.

A bilingual or even multilingual upbringing can certainly

be confusing. For a while, young bilingual children may speak several languages in the same conversation or sentence, but the important point is that they speak as fluently as any other child.

Anyone who really knows about a bilingual upbringing knows that it is very unlikely to cause language delay. Look closely at youngsters with speech delay, and you'll find they don't say much in any language. The message is that if you think your twins have a language difficulty, get a proper assessment (including a hearing check), however many languages they are exposed to.

Chapter Eleven
PRE-SCHOOL TWINS

I worried so much about sending them to playgroup. Would they be happy? They were together, but would they miss me? Would they each make friends? While I fretted, they were blissfully and busily happy almost all the time. The only time they were miserable was when I was late because the car broke down.

The pre-school years cover the ages of about three to five years. It is a delightful time that many parents say brings the best of both worlds. Children are still very close to their mothers at this age, but they are growing up and becoming more biddable. Most pre-schoolers get the chance of going to playgroup or nursery school for up to twenty hours a week. This brings many opportunities for new experiences, but there are some things to bear in mind:

- Multiples should be prioritised for pre-school and nursery education, but the level of provision varies around the country. There is a huge patchwork of public and private provision which affects what your family can be offered.
- However good the local pre-school facilities are, parents continue to be the main educators of children at this age.
- Pre-school twins still need a lot of adult time and attention – again, this means yours. That's something which is still in short supply, particularly if you are returning to work.
- During the pre-school years, many twins begin to be aware of their twinship and therefore of being different from most other children, who are singletons. This is at least partly because adults and other children treat them as unusual.

- This can result in twins being lumped together, which often marks the beginning of a lifelong battle for each child to be valued for himself.

I was so disappointed that, after three years of doing our best to help Leah and Amber develop individuality, our efforts were completely undermined by a couple of mornings at playgroup. The leader obviously treated them as one and by the end of their second session the children were calling them 'Twins' instead of using their names.

- Unfortunately, many playgroups and nurseries are still inexperienced in the issues concerning multiple-birth children. Those that are may have views that don't coincide with yours. Be extra vigilant to make sure your children get the best out of their pre-school.
- The more you make of the pre-school years, the better prepared your children will be for their school career and the better they will probably do in both language and behaviour.

· *Pre-school Education* ·

Obviously, playgroups and nurseries give children the chance to get out of the house and away from their parents (unless they happen to be playgroup leaders). If nothing else, this teaches youngsters about separation, which is an important experience for many children, especially if they are rarely looked after by anyone other than Mum.

Pre-school also gives young children exposure to a slightly more structured environment, which is good preparation for 'big school'. At this age, children love to conform, which makes it a great time to introduce routine.

Pre-school allows children to play with toys they don't have at home and to experiment with a variety of new materials. For twins and other multiples, it provides vital opportunities for creative play, such as finger-painting, which they may not get in their own homes because the mess would be hard to handle in the house. It also reinforces the enjoyment of singing, saying rhymes, listening to stories and looking at books, all of which are important in developing language and learning to read. This is the time when a young child's literacy and love of books, as well as basic skills in writing and number, are established.

Play is actually a serious business, as educationalists emphasise. Take role play. As well as being good all-round fun, dressing up and taking on different roles enables a child to experience different situations and experiment with them. Through all kinds of play, a child learns about his environment. Twins education expert and former headteacher Pat Preedy, who is Tamba's education research consultant, points out: 'Remember, play is not something that is given as a reward after work. Through play, the child builds firm foundations for later learning. Children who have difficulties with learning have often had impoverished play experiences.' She also adds that it is important for a child to learn sustained play, instead of flitting from one activity to another. This is something a number of twins are prone to do, perhaps because they are used to being distracted and interrupted.

The way a child tackles tasks is important too. Discussing an activity beforehand and afterwards is vital to taking learning forward. The child who learns to 'plan, do and review' acquires the ability to focus and stay on track, clearly a valuable life-skill.

Playgroups and nurseries also teach children elementary social skills, such as taking turns, something multiples especially need to acquire. Children aged three or more are usually ready to make friends outside the family and pre-school play provides good opportunities for mixing and playing alongside another child other than his own twin.

· *Which Pre-school?* ·

Provision varies from area to area. At one extreme there may be the chance of just a couple of two-hour sessions a week for your children at a playgroup in a local church hall, while at the other end of the spectrum there may be enough nursery places, attached to primary schools, for all children of pre-school age.

Most suburban areas fall somewhere in the middle, with many playgroups (which you have to pay for) offering a variety of hours and perhaps two or more state-run nursery schools with a long list of children waiting for spaces for sessions. These are usually held every morning (or afternoon) of the week, each session lasting two and a half hours.

In some areas, all pre-school children eventually get a nursery place, but perhaps only for one term just before they start primary school – equitable maybe, but of limited use. If you are thinking ahead to strategies for primary school entry, one thing to realise now is that there's no such thing as a 'feeder' nursery for a particular school. The exceptions are in the private sector and with certain religious schools.

You may be able to get your twins or triplets into a nursery school a term or two ahead of most singletons if you can convince the authorities that they have special needs. For example, you might emphasise the greater need they have to acquire social skills, or you could point out any learning or language difficulties they may already have. Equally, though, multiples may be ready later than singletons, for instance because they were premature. A developmental assessment (ask your family doctor) could back up your request, and you can also ask Tamba for assistance. Unfortunately, showing that your children desperately need nursery does not make vacancies materialise. There aren't enough places, and the more multiples you have the greater the problem.

Look around at what is available. It ought to be nearby, not only to make it easy for you, but to enable your children to see their friends socially outside the playgroup, at birthday parties and so on.

Start your search early – no later than their second birthday and possibly much earlier – even if they cannot start until they are nearly three years old. Because you have more than one child, you have more decisions to make. You need more places too, so get their names down in plenty of time. It is not much good discovering that the ideal playgroup can accommodate only one of your triplets.

Don't be embarrassed about visiting lots of playgroups to get a feel for what is on offer. There are obvious things you'll need to know, like the cost and the number and length of sessions available (is each one long enough for you to get to the shops and back, for instance?). But you could also ask more searching questions:

1 How structured are the sessions? Are children allowed to get on with their choice of activity or are they shepherded at predetermined times from one thing to the next? Is there any progression? For instance, are the older children (rising-fives) treated separately for part of the session, in preparation for school? If so, are twins automatically in the same group? This may be fine for many multiples, but you have to decide what will be best for yours.

2 How is discipline achieved? Is it based just on verbal warnings, or is any exclusion or 'time out' meted out as punishment?

3 Does the playgroup leader or nursery teacher have any experience of multiples? Probably not, but this is a good opening question for introducing the subject. Perhaps the teacher has taught very few multiples, but has had literature from Tamba or is planning to attend a course or

study day. Although experience is vital, the right attitude is more important. Watch out for sweeping statements such as 'All twins are like that.' In reality, there are very few areas in which all twins are alike.

4   Check out the parents' rota – almost all playgroups have one, while nurseries don't normally count on parental help. Is a mother of triplets expected to help out three times as often? Clearly, you may have three times the usual number of children, but there's still only one of you and you should not be roped into doing more than other parents.

5   If you are going to send both (or all) of your children to the same playgroup, ask about a bulk discount on fees. You're unlikely to get one, but it does no harm to ask.

6   Don't forget to ask yourself whether you like the atmosphere of the playgroup. This may prove to be more important to you and your children than some of the other factors.

· *Together or Apart?* ·

Playgroup could give you an ideal opportunity to spend a little regular protected time with each child on her own, so should you send your twins together or not? This may be the first occasion you have to consider the question of separation, but it's an issue that will crop up again and again during your children's school careers.

It is impossible to say which option is better for twins in the long term. The research just has not been done, and in any case the best course of action depends on your family. Twins who show a little language delay or behaviour problems may benefit from separate playgroups, for instance, but if they have never been separated, they are likely to find this traumatic.

Sometimes only one twin is ready for playgroup, just as one may be out of nappies before the other. It is usually right to send that child on ahead. Holding her back could be wrong – a good example of equal treatment being unfair. Besides, sending her to playgroup may encourage her brother to become dry very soon.

If you have triplets or more, your options as well as your time will be more limited, but with twins there is usually some leeway. Here are some options:

1 You send your children to the same playgroup on different days. In this way they will both benefit from similar experiences and learn about separation not only from you but from each other. By attending on different days, your twins are also less likely to be mistaken for each other – in theory, anyway! On the other hand, this gives you little or no time on your own and the child who is at home on a particular day may feel very left out unless you make an effort to do something with him.

   For nearly half a term, James went on Mondays and Wednesdays, while Ben went on Tuesdays and Thursdays. Whoever was at home with me moped around and didn't really settle to anything, while I got increasingly harassed. It was my health visitor who pointed out that I was making a rod for my own back.

2 They attend separate playgroups altogether. This gives you more time to yourself and the twins benefit from the maximum number of sessions available. If they are ready and happy to be apart, this will work well, but if not they could view this enforced separation as a punishment or ordeal. Consider the logistics as well. Ferrying them to different destinations can be hard, especially if you have other children too.

3 You send them together. The children learn about

separation from you without the trauma of breaking away from each other. Do watch how the playgroup staff and helpers treat your twins. You may find them being constantly compared, confused or treated as a single unit. Other young children are often very good at knowing who is who, even with identicals, but if grown-ups constantly refer to your children as 'the twins' it will rub off.

I felt I could tell off the leader gently but it was a losing battle when all the other kids talked about 'the twins'. Even though they always knew which was which, it was as if they couldn't be bothered, and that wasn't healthy, in my opinion.

4   A solution that works well for some parents is sending twins separately for one or two sessions a week, and together the rest of the time. However, this option leaves you having to entertain the one who is not at playgroup. Bear in mind that it also gives playgroup leaders occasional scope for confusion; for example, 'You did a lovely picture yesterday, Harry. Or was that Jack?' Other children can get confused too.

5   With nursery school there are fewer options, though you may be able to send one twin to morning sessions and the other in the afternoon. Timing during the lunch period can be a little tight, but this arrangement works well for some.

My mother had the girls separately. She'd have one in the morning and the other in the afternoon, which was nice for them and for her. In fact, she could really only manage one of my daughters at a time so it was an ideal arrangement for all concerned, provided I came back from work at lunchtime and gave her a hand.

As a parent, you'll know whether your children would be

better off together or not, and what fits in best with your lifestyle. Don't flog yourself with separate playgroups for each child if it makes things too hard. When your twins get home from each session, they need Mum to be her cheerful, energetic best, not a limp rag.

· *When Your Children are at Pre-school* ·

As a parent, there are many things you can do to help your twins or triplets get the most from playgroup or nursery:

- Twins shouldn't have to do everything together. Co-operation may make some things happen, but it can also hinder learning and the development of their individuality. They also need to learn the skill of co-operating with other children, not just each other.

  So if your children aren't already placed in separate groups within the nursery, ask if they could be. Some teachers put them together 'to help them settle in', then forget all about separating them later. In reality, few twins need to sit side by side the whole time – even pairs who are very dependent on each other are usually happy as long as each knows where the other is.
- Help the staff and other parents to distinguish between your children. Present your multiples as individuals. Use different clothing (hairstyles too if you can) so that playgroup and nursery staff can tell your twins apart at a glance. Name labels or badges can help, but remove them promptly on leaving playgroup. I'm wary of jumpers (or gym bags and lunch-boxes) emblazoned with names as these can be a security hazard, since any stranger will know what they're called.
- Impress on staff the need to call your children by name, and ask them also to encourage the other children to do the

same. Ensure that you set a good example yourself.

I knew I'd won when one of the other mothers on the parents' rota spent two mornings helping before she even realised Alex and Kim were related. The fact that they were each dressed very differently certainly helped.

- Dress children for mess: they will get filthy by the end of each session and you may flip if your twins are covered in flour and face paint when you pick them up. If they wear clothes that don't matter, you will feel a lot better. Wet wipes kept in the car or buggy help deal with sticky hands. (A couple of plastic carrier bags in the boot to transport still-wet works of art are also a good idea.)
- When you pick them up, ask each child how his day went. Twins rarely have any privacy. They also need to know you are interested in them as individuals. So don't let one of them spill the beans to you about his twin's news, no matter how keen he is.
- Similarly, if you want to know if Becky cried when you left, or was banished to the corner for any misdemeanours, best ask an adult rather than her brother Sam. Besides, you may get a pack of lies: twins sometimes enjoy telling tall tales.
- Try to appreciate their efforts, be they lopsided fairy cakes or pasta pictures. It is important to make the right noises, even though you will have twice as many of these to take home as the other mums and the novelty does wear off.
- If your twins are very different in ability, try to avoid negative comparisons. One child's painting may look somewhat sad next to his twin's competent self-portrait, but you can always find something positive to say, such as 'I really like that colour.' One mother opted for: 'That's a great style, Gregory – I think it might even be cubist.'
- When it is your turn to help out, keep in the background, but take the opportunity to watch your children during the

session. You may be surprised by how differently they behave at playgroup. On the other hand, it may be just like it is at home. One mother of triplets commented that at playgroup hers just functioned as a pack for months, roaming together with hardly any interaction with other children. This can also be true of quads and more.

- When they start making friends, be prepared for plenty of cries of ''S not fair!' One of your children may well be invited out more than his twin, at least to begin with. When one is asked round to tea at a friend's, don't ask if his twin can come too. Instead, try to make that time more interesting for the one who has not been invited. Do something nice, just the two of you. There's a whole different world out there when you've only got one child in tow. Go swimming, perhaps, since that's hard with two children. Or else ask another little friend round to your place for him to play with while his twin is out. Eventually he'll be asked out too, and the score usually evens up. It doesn't always, but then life is unfair.

· *Preparing for 'Big School'* ·

Whether your children are at playgroup or nursery school, or at home with you, the pre-school years are vital in terms of preparing them for primary school and the rest of their scholastic career. In general, the more you do to promote your twins' individualities and identities now at this stage, the easier their schooldays will be.

- Forget techniques such as cramming, rote learning or other methods to speed up learning. These are not so much learning methods as party pieces and, however impressed other mums may be, they probably won't help your children at all.

- Encourage each child to learn to concentrate, whether it is on a book, a jigsaw or a construction toy, for five to ten minutes at a time despite the presence of his twin. This is desperately difficult for many twins to learn because they are so used to interfering with each other's activities.
- Teach them to take turns. This is another skill that's vital for success in the classroom and the playground, one you can teach quite simply with almost any daily activities.
- Help them communicate. As mentioned in the previous chapter, twins are often ace at interrupting. Some need to be taught to slow down and speak at an appropriate pace, so that people can understand them.
- Encourage your children to talk without shouting. I know it's hard in a household full of noisy youngsters, and you are likely to be shouting much of the time too, if only to make yourself heard above the twin-din, but it's worth a try.
- Extend their vocabulary and language skills as best you can. This means talking to each child clearly, slowly enough and appropriately (with actions that match what you are saying to that child). Remember to make eye contact with the one you are addressing.
- Make books fun. Borrow a variety from the library. Your youngsters can have their own tickets from an early age (incidentally, there are often no fines payable on children's tickets) and will enjoy the magic of 'turning them into books' at the borrowing desk. Talk about the books you liked or have enjoyed, and read to them. It is still helpful to read to each twin separately if you can, but a bedtime story read together is better than none at all.
- Set a good example: households where adults enjoy reading tend to nurture youngsters who do too. Encourage your twins to talk and think about things. You could ask questions such as 'Why do you think that bus is going so slowly now that it is raining?' If you don't know the answer

to something they ask, resolve (at least occasionally) to look it up and let them know what it is. It will be ages before they are able to use encyclopaedias or the internet themselves, but that's not the point – the aim is to encourage enquiring minds and show that the answers can be found if one looks.

- Teach your children how to dress themselves. This applies to singletons too, though with twins it is even more tempting (and a lot faster) to dress them yourself, but they need to learn to do it themselves. Watch out for twins who dress each other: in a boy-girl pair, the girl will sometimes dress her brother.

- Let each have a little privacy from his twin whenever possible. Most twins share a bedroom at this age, but they needn't always both play in it at the same time. If they move into separate bedrooms, sometimes an extra bed, or a mattress on the floor, can help as there may be times when they like to sleep in the same room.

- Increase one-to-one contact if you can, with separate outings, for example.

- As in earlier years, avoid labelling or creating artificial distinctions between them.

- Treat your child in a way that is appropriate for his age. Your twins are growing up, but it is often hard for a parent to notice it, especially when their pre-school children are still in a buggy, or are very cute, as is often the case with multiples.

- Be positive about school. If you didn't enjoy your own schooldays, either keep quiet about it, or be selective about what you say. 'I didn't like my school-bag because it was brown' is less alarming than the fact that you were scared stiff of the headteacher.

Finally, prepare yourself for the time when your children will go off to school for several hours every day, leaving you, perhaps for the first time since their birth, with the luxury of deciding what to do – whether it is returning to work with a merchant bank or learning to arrange flowers. Faced with the all-consuming demands of rearing twins or more, you may have lost touch with some of the things that matter to you. If you have, the start of term in September may be something of a milestone, giving you the chance to give some thought to yourself. But life can suddenly feel a little empty when your 'babies' begin at primary school. Strangely enough, it is sometimes mums who have always had their own careers who feel most bereft when their twins start school.

Chapter Twelve

PRIMARY SCHOOL

My daughters greeted me outside the classroom, their cheeks glowing and their eyes like saucers. They were burning to tell me their latest discovery – that they like fish fingers.

One of the most exciting aspects of having twins start school is seeing them enjoy new experiences, and sharing these enthusiastically with you. Primary school is a wonderful time, full of opportunities for making friends and learning new skills, before homework and exams become all-consuming. But there can be hiccups. Every year Tamba receives an increasing number of requests for help with twins at primary school and beyond.

Parents occasionally have concerns about their twins' education because of earlier problems with prematurity or growth retardation, or perhaps because one of them spent time in special care as a baby. Past medical or physical disorders can sometimes affect a youngster's school career. Even when they don't, it can be hard to believe that all will be well if they had a wobbly start in life. Understandably, some parents continue to have anxieties about their once-sickly offspring for many years.

How will your twins fare? Several research projects have looked at the performance of multiples at primary school. Early large-scale studies came from Australia, from a nationwide study which began in 1985, and also from the La Trobe University Twin Study, which, starting in 1978, looked at how twins progressed in terms of behaviour and skills both at home and at school.

Now newer work has shed more light on how twins do at primary school in the UK. As headteacher at Knowle Infant School in the Midlands, Pat Preedy began her research into twins at school when, in 1992, she had a record nine sets of twins in her nursery and reception classes. Spurred on by Tamba, she then carried out a national survey of several thousand schools and how they cope with multiples, from twins to quins. Later in this chapter you'll find more about Pat Preedy's findings (and those of others) which are relevant to parents. You may also like to look at the excellent twin education website *www.twinsandmultiples.org* authored by Pat Preedy and David Hay (see page 372) and launched in 2001. Aimed at parents and professionals around the world, it covers a huge range of issues that affect multiples at school.

One thing you may need to decide is when to start school. When children are born very premature, it can make more sense for them to begin their formal education based on their due date, not the date they were born. Twins due in October, say, could find themselves embarking on their school careers a whole year earlier if they were born eight weeks early, and this isn't always in their interests. Education authorities tend to interpret rules strictly and may tell you that there is no choice. However, if you have a good case then Tamba may be able to help.

· *Together or Apart?* ·

Whether or not twins should be put in the same class at school is not necessarily the most crucial issue where their education is concerned, but it has huge practical implications. Plus you have to consider it early. Most parents have some say in this, though circumstances can limit the choice if:

• one of your twins has special needs

- you have a boy-girl pair and you intend to educate them in the independent sector (where schools are still often segregated by sex even at the pre-prep stage)
- you live in a small rural community.

As one parent says:

> *Before we moved here, we were told it was county policy to split twins up and put them in separate classes within a school, but when we investigated we found that all three local primary schools had only one intake. Separating our two girls would have involved different schools, with all the attendant problems of that, and we couldn't have coped.*

More about 'policy' later, but first a look at some of the potential advantages and disadvantages of each choice. Twins often gain a lot from each other's support. When they start school in the same class, they can find it easier than a singleton to be away from home and parents Their school-work can benefit from an element of competition. On the other hand, they may distract each other, especially when they're sitting close together, and both concentration and behaviour can suffer. They may check on each other constantly, or even copy work. Even when they don't cheat, teachers sometimes think they have.

When things go wrong, twins may collude or blame each other. Teachers can become thoroughly confused, especially with identical twins, and often with same-sex fraternal twins too. If this happens, then neither twin may get the learning she needs. When one twin is dominant, the other may be so dependent that she seems unable to work or make her own friends.

There can be problems when the twins are very different in ability, and one always trails behind. Inevitably, teachers will then make comparisons, and these are bound to flatter one child at the expense of her twin. This may become even more common now that testing is so prevalent, even at primary level. Bear in mind too that only one child in each class can ever come first, which can seem hugely unfair to twins, especially when they are of equal ability.

Putting twins into separate classes may seem ideal. After all, they can be themselves, and may make their own friends more easily (though they will be together in the playground). In class, each will be able to progress at her own pace, which is particularly important when there are differences in ability (even MZ twins can have very different learning styles). They will undoubtedly enjoy more privacy, something twins rarely have. Children may behave better without the constant stimulus and competition of their twin. Teachers will certainly be less confused, and staff may get to know each twin far better when they have no choice but to relate to each as an individual. On the other hand, your children are bound to compare their teachers, their classrooms, and the reading-books they take home. Perhaps most important of all, starting school is a major life event – will your children need each other?

So, together or apart? No single answer is right for every family and it is a question of which is more likely to bring out the best in your twins. Putting them in separate classes isn't a cure-all, even though many parents think it will be. After all, children still spend more of their time at home than they do in class, even during term-time. In deciding what suits your children, you should take two main factors into account: the twins' relative abilities and their relationship with each other.

If you have a boy-girl pair, teachers will have few problems telling them apart, but a potential difficulty is that girls are often more advanced, especially in language, and may take charge in class (she may do her twin's work for him too).

If one twin is dominant, the dependent one may benefit

from being in a separate class (or even a different school), though the dominant one may find it hard being on his own to begin with.

Do your twins function well independently? If so, separation is less of an issue, but if one tends to opt out of activities, they may both benefit from being apart.

Are there obvious physical differences between them? A twin who is less confident because he is shorter, less healthy or less co-ordinated than his brother may improve in self-esteem once out of his twin's shadow.

Consider how competitive they are. Does each concentrate well or are they distracted by each other? Sometimes like-minded twins can be a combustible mixture.

What else is going on in the family – a divorce or a house move? At difficult times, twins can get a lot of comfort from being together, so perhaps a separation could be postponed.

Many twins starting school have rarely been apart, as Pat Preedy's work confirms. Some pairs may have been separated only when some unpleasant incident has occurred, for instance when one of them has had to go into hospital.

Have your twins been away from home already, for instance at nursery? How often and for how long are they normally apart? Perhaps they spend weekends with grand-parents separately. What are their perceptions of being apart: fun or punishment? Do they like each other's company? It is worth considering all these points. You won't necessarily do something just because the youngsters suggest it, but their views ought to be taken into account. Pat Preedy's research uncovered the worrying fact that the adults involved often don't discuss with multiples how the children themselves feel. Following on from this, she and Mary Lowe of Tamba produced the book *Multiple Voices* to illustrate the views and opinions of twins, triplets and more.

For those of you still undecided on this issue, there's a very useful checklist on *www.twinsandmultiples.org*.

Triplets and more

If you want your triplets to be in different classes, how can you do this? A few schools may have three parallel classes, but most just aren't big enough. Putting the closer pair together in one class can work, although the third one may feel left out on her own. For some triplet families, a reasonable solution is to separate the one who is of different gender; another is to put a non-identical pair together. You may prefer two or even three different schools, but bear in mind the extra effort involved, especially if they have different term-times. Or, even worse, the same day for the end-of-term play.

Actually I enjoyed having the kids at home at different times in half-terms and holidays. It didn't happen often, but when it did it meant special days with just one or two of my triplets instead of the whole trio.

If they will be separated at school, but haven't spent much time apart so far, it can be useful to have a planned programme of separate outings and activities for at least a few months before the start of term.

On the other hand, there's no reason why placing all your triplets (or quads) in the same class will not work, especially if they are in different groups within the class. Triplets can function well in the same class and some teachers see advantages in it. They're more likely to understand the trio from the family's point of view, and to appreciate the dynamics of their relationships. A dedicated (and preferably experienced) teacher can be very upbeat about the challenge.

It is just that the more children you have, the fewer your options. A school may even refuse to give you places for all three 'on principle': it has been known for headteachers to believe they cannot possibly make that many places available to just one family. But you do have the right to appeal against decisions you believe are not in your children's best interests.

School policies

Some schools have a policy on twins, usually to separate them in class (or, less often, to place them together) regardless of the circumstances. If the school's prevailing policy happens to fit in with what you wanted for your children anyway, that's fine. If not, you can challenge it. Tamba can advise parents on this and may be able to write a letter to support your point of view.

But at heart it's wrong for schools to have a fixed strategy. As those with expertise in educating multiples sometimes say, the best policy is no policy – or, rather, no rigid policy. In these days of written policies on everything, a school should have some written acknowledgement of the fact that twins and multiples are a special case. Ideally the policy should enshrine the right of multiples to be educated on their own merits. Otherwise, a blanket ruling may just be a cover for not thinking properly about the issues. There is a framework policy for schools on *www.twinsandmultiples.org* which your children's school may like to adapt.

In practice

What happens where there is no firm policy on multiples? Decisions are usually made collectively by headteachers, class teachers and parents. If nobody asks for your opinion, give it anyway. Sometimes a decision is made to keep twins and more together on somewhat arbitrary grounds, for instance date of birth!

In practice, most twins start primary school in the same class. Preedy's research showed that twice as many of them were together as were apart at primary level. Many twins settle in better at big school if they know they won't be separated. In this way they can learn to become independent of you without having to be apart from each other at the same time.

This can make a mum feel left out:

On the first day, they went off together into the classroom without so much as a backward glance, while I stood there with a great big lump in my throat.

If your twins are in the same class, it is usually best for them to be placed in separate groups within the class to avoid being lumped together, distracting each other or collaborating when they should be working independently.

Sam and Robert were seated side by side in their new school, but they never settled because they were constantly fighting instead of getting on with it. The teacher called me in to say she was having terrible trouble with my boys and what did I think was the matter – was there a problem at home? And I had to explain to her that it was really her doing. They were no trouble at all when they were placed at separate tables and in fact soon outperformed all the other children in the class! I was bursting with pride when I realised what they were capable of achieving.

The separate/apart decision needs to be revisited, usually many times. During their primary school careers, many twins end up in different classes, with a decision to separate them being taken at the end of the reception year, or later. Some pairs go their separate ways at the age of seven. One big pitfall: if one child stays with his original class and the other goes to a different one, leaving his friends as well as his twin could be a big wrench. He may find it an uphill struggle to start all over again with a new group, while his twin sails calmly on.

When they are placed in different classes, it can be helpful for each to see the other one's classroom, so that he can picture where his twin will spend most of the day. If they are at different schools, this can be even more important.

Taking stock

No decision you make should be truly irreversible: you don't always know at the time what is right, and parenting as a whole is a huge experiment. It is a good idea to reappraise progress every so often, possibly at the end of the school year, and whenever else you or the teachers think it advisable. The important thing is to be flexible. It doesn't really matter whether your children are together or apart, as long as they are happy and making good progress. And that depends a lot on the attitudes towards them at school and at home.

Teachers and twins

Thanks to the efforts of Tamba, MBF and the families of twins themselves, there is increasing awareness of the issues of multiples at school, but even so some professionals remain unenlightened. Every teacher in the UK is likely to have at least a set of twins to teach, yet formal training for teachers rarely covers this area.

Some teachers just generalise from the previous set of twins they taught, but of course there is no such thing as 'typical twins'. A few twins are hardly aware of each other, while others are intimately inter-reliant and others still fight non-stop in class (not yours, you hope . . .).

At the start of the school year, you may not know where your children's teachers stand. The staff will want to do their best for your twins and chances are they will be open-minded. I have certainly found this, and my own twins have had some teachers of the highest calibre. However, I think it's best not to assume that all teachers are well versed in handling multiples. For instance, one or two parents have discovered that their twins have had just one combined baseline assessment between them. Such situations could perhaps be avoided by trying to find out early in the school year how a teacher handles twins in class.

Many teachers are eager and willing to know more, and we parents too are all learning constantly. Everyone involved, whether parents or teachers, should be humble enough at least to listen to one another. In your dealings with your twins' teachers, co-operation rather than confrontation is the best strategy. Keep lines of communication open by meeting often. This also ensures that you know what's going on in class.

There's a lot more that schools could do to help multiples, and your children's school may like to know about the educational opportunities provided by Tamba. Tamba also produces an excellent general leaflet for schools. As a starter, you could give one to your twins' teachers.

· *How Multiples Do at School* ·

Are problems any more common in twins? There are no consistent differences between singletons and multiples in intelligence, or in maths and other subjects, but Australian research strongly suggests that reading is an issue, especially for boys. While the Australian work showed that most twins have no problems, it highlighted the suspicion that difficulties at school might be more likely in:

- identical (MZ) twins
- male twins
- those with a sibling only two to three years older

- those who speak a language other than English at home
- those born premature or who had a lot of early medical problems.

There is some controversy about how twins perform at school, and new evidence from the UK indicates that they do no worse than singletons, so in itself twinning does not seem to be a handicap in terms of achievement.

The PIPS (Performance Indicators in Primary Schools) project was developed by Professor Peter Tymms at Durham to focus on the progress children make in school relative to their starting point at school entry. This is a measure of the value added by education, as it were. In this age of league tables, some schools have consistently more impressive results, but it could be partly because they select more able or more privileged pupils. In other words, to know how well a school performs, and how well a child does, you need to know the level at which each child started, and then assess progress relative to that. PIPS compares children at the same starting point and looks at where they were expected to finish. If children achieve more than expected, then this is the value added.

PIPS is now used widely in schools to make baseline assessments at school entry. Using material that is fun for children, it evaluates each child's non-verbal ability, picture vocabulary and the amount of educational input a child gets at home. Its uses extend far beyond twin issues. However, within a large sample Peter Tymms and Pat Preedy identified twins and multiples, and came up with some encouraging conclusions. In a nutshell, twins, triplets and more don't seem to be disadvantaged compared with singletons when they start primary school. They probably do just as well as singletons in their first year at school. Moreover, they don't differ appreciably from singletons in 'early literacy' scores (pre-reading skills), though they may have a slight reading delay which soon evens out.

These findings conflict with a lot of the earlier Australian work, but the studies looked at different populations at different times, and there could be cultural differences too. In 1990s Britain there could have been greater awareness of twins' issues. It could also be relevant that the recent increase in multiple births is largely amongst women over 35, who are often more advantaged and educated to a higher level than younger mothers.

One reassuring finding from the British research is that multiples are good at early language or pre-reading skills. A possible explanation is that, whatever happens later, twins and higher-order multiples start with the same potential for language and reading as singletons. It's then up to parents and teachers to bring out the best in them.

· *Possible Problems at School* ·

This doesn't mean that your twins will have problems, but even so it's wise to be aware of areas where they can crop up. When there are difficulties, it's tempting to assume fatalistically that they will grow out of whatever it is, or that it has happened simply because they are twins. Occasionally both are true, but it's good to know when you need to take action.

Reading

Many children have trouble reading. Some learn later than others, some read inaccurately, others read accurately but with poor understanding, and a few seem competent but just don't enjoy it much.

Reading difficulties may improve in time, but they don't always. If one of your twins seems to have trouble, it is worth doing something about it early on in his school career, as so much depends on being able to read well. You need to liaise closely with the teacher and may also need the advice of an educational psychologist. It is also worth checking your child's eyesight.

Sometimes all you need to do as a parent is help with reading at home. If you do, make sure that your child learns to read accurately. Don't just move your finger under the text: twins tend to rush and may not understand, so take it slowly and ask your child casual but interesting questions to check his comprehension.

Learning support is sometimes necessary. This usually takes place at school, but wherever it is, you need to co-operate closely with the teacher. There is more about special educational needs in Chapter 15.

If both children need asssistance, make sure each gets his full quota, not half what a singleton would receive. If only one of your children is poor at reading, help him accept this calmly. It is hard to be different from (especially less good than) your twin when the whole world expects you to be just the same. Teach him to see that no two people are the same at everything, whether it is football or reading. It's tricky striking the right balance, but don't ignore the achievements of the more able twin!

Bad behaviour

Problems aren't inevitable here either, but bad behaviour can be a major issue at school as well as at home. It may be linked with language and reading problems, but this isn't always the case. Very able children often misbehave because they are bored, and because their intellectual abilities outstrip their social skills – a matter of IQ versus emotional intelligence. According to teachers and parents of twins, fighting and competing seem to cause most upheaval.

Fighting and aggressive behaviour

Fighting, covered in Chapter 10, is more common in twins, especially boys of primary-school age.

> *I thought everything was fine because they'd become so settled at home. But one of the other kids in their class informed me that they were always hitting each other at playtime. It was true, as I discovered from many subsequent meetings with their teacher. I actually began to dread seeing her outside the school at three-thirty and feared that she was scanning the horizon for me in order to lodge yet another complaint.*

Often the children's aggression is seen only within the twinship: they may kick each other mercilessly at the slightest provocation, yet not lay a finger on other children.

One of the difficulties is trying to unravel what happened at school. This can be hard enough for a teacher to sort out even at the time of the incident. By the time your twins come out of school in the afternoon, you'll get their versions of events – with economy of truth as well as simultaneously and at full blast. You may not have a hope of finding out who started it or why, but that doesn't really matter. I suggest you give up the struggle and concentrate on what matters: teaching the children that fighting gets them nowhere.

On the whole, a school is best equipped to deal with school-based problems, but schools need full parental support. In handling twins who fight, it helps to:

- keep them constantly occupied
- help them make their own friends
- reward good behaviour
- ensure that fighting results in loss of privileges (and no melting when they hug you sweetly two minutes after the latest brawl).

A little distance between warring twins can also work wonders. This may be a good opportunity for more separate outings, or for separate bedrooms if you can arrange it. Often one twin is aggressive because he feels put upon, left behind or inferior in some way. If so, building his self-esteem could dramatically reduce his tendency to outbursts of violence or angry frustration.

Competition

This may be another facet of the same problem – rivalry. It can also be, like fighting, an expression of a need for attention. Some competition is healthy: one twin may set standards that the other strives to match.

> *My two boys are like two peas in a pod in looks and academic work. In the same class they were thought to be a potential disaster because of fighting, but there was no choice at the local school, which only had one intake. However, it worked out really well. They egg each other on so that they are both at the top of the class (jointly because their marks are identical). They are more than a year ahead in maths and many other subjects. Their older sister is just as bright but doesn't often achieve as much. Being a singleton, perhaps she just doesn't have that competitive edge.*

But competition can also mean lack of care, rushed work, careless mistakes, interruptions in class, finishing sentences for each other – and seriously getting on the teacher's nerves if the twins are in the same class.

They may also compete for friends and in sports. If they are in different school houses, on sports day one may be elated while his twin is miserable.

> *I knew they were each capable of good work, but they were so busy checking on each other's progress (and trying to finish first) even*

when they weren't in close proximity in class. I think they hardly ever achieved what they could have. If I placed the girls where they couldn't see each other, they'd still turn around and crane their necks . . .

Some teachers find that twins are constantly aware of each other both in class and out. If this becomes disruptive and wastes teaching time, it may be better to separate them into two different classes. Having done this, each twin may still need to know where the other one is. Often a twin finds it reassuring to become familiar with his twin's classroom too.

· *Comparisons between Twins* ·

It's natural to compare, and when there is another child of exactly the same age the temptation becomes irresistible. On some levels it is useful: you can tell that Natalie has a fever because her forehead feels so much hotter than Lorraine's, for example.

Most of the time it is less helpful. Strangely, one often compares twins' abilities when the differences between them are actually minute, which magnifies their importance out of all proportion. It is common for one twin to be thought less able, or even slow, when in reality he is very like his twin. It is not unknown for a difference of two percentage points in a maths test to result in a nasty punch-up.

Most parents cherish their twins' differences, which makes it doubly hard to avoid comparisons. But comparisons can seriously affect the children's own perceptions, expectations and ambitions, and could critically injure the confidence of one of them. Another danger is that, like labels, comparisons are sometimes wrong. For now, Ruth may be the better reader, but a few weeks later Becky might have taken off.

Different abilities

A more able child can easily outshine his twin's efforts. On the other hand, sometimes he may help him so often that differences in ability go unnoticed for some time, until perhaps there's a classroom test.

It becomes very difficult for parents when there are real differences in ability or performance. If one child achieves more, the other by definition achieves less. If one is a winner, the other must be the loser. There is no middle ground. We say we all love our children equally, but there is no doubt that some families – university lecturers' and musicians' families are two obvious examples – put a very high premium on certain talents and achievements.

It is important to find something that the less academic child is good at, and to celebrate his achievements. Otherwise self-esteem can become seriously low. Sometimes twins can usefully be channelled into different activities, especially in a choice of sport or musical instrument, but one mustn't invent differences in interests or ignore the children's own preferences and talents. Perhaps they really do both want to learn the violin, play football or go to Brownies. It might, paradoxically, be better for their development as individuals to let them both do the same activities. But if you can manage it, it is sometimes beneficial for the children to do them separately from one other.

· *The Joys* ·

Like most parenting books, this one concentrates on the demands of raising a family. But twins starting at primary school can bring great joy to their parents and it is worth pausing to enjoy the fun and count the advantages. Here are some parents' comments:

I went back to work. Life was finally normal again.

I was thrilled that we'd actually got to this stage. When they were tiny and premature there were days when it seemed impossible.

The best thing? Without doubt it is the first school photo. Other parents just get a picture of one child, but I had one taken of them together, their faces scrubbed, their eyes shiny, their ties wonky as usual.

They love school and have rushed off happily every morning almost without exception. But equally they're always thrilled to see me in the playground when they come out. Every afternoon I'm practically knocked over as they race to greet me with a double helping of hugs and cuddles. I know other mothers envy me too.

They are making new friends. Twins seem popular with other children, and none of the kids has trouble telling them apart.

Two lots of artwork to treasure. I even had some of their paintings framed. They look wonderful hanging side by side.

And before long you too will have many delicious moments to cherish.

· *What Parents Can Do* ·

Help each child look and feel like an individual. This is especially important for single-sex pairs, but school uniforms don't help. Girls (and some boys) can have different hairstyles. It is often possible to customise school uniform, for example:

- pinafore for one, skirt for the other
- different styles of jumper

- different shades of grey trousers or skirts
- different shoes, overcoats and school-bags.

In one school, one boy was allowed to wear the old-style school tie while his twin had the newer type. Different clothing is also an aid to safety.

- Don't refer to your children as 'the twins' or 'the triplets' if you can help it. If you need a collective noun, call them 'my/the children'.
- Be alert for teachers and anyone else who treats them as one unit. You can point out gently that this is hurtful or unsettling for the children. One mother was most distressed to find the teacher referred to her two as Pinky and Perky, and soon, unfortunately, their classmates did the same.
- Encourage each child to take in his own notes or messages for the teacher, dinner money, etc., in separate envelopes. Otherwise some pairs may allot roles and insist that, for example, 'Only Kim takes notes for the school office.'
- Ask your children every so often whether the teacher gets them mixed up. You might be surprised to hear that some twins get inaccurate educational assessments because staff cannot reliably tell them apart.
- Does one child usually tell you the other's news? Encourage each twin to talk to you in turn about her day at school. Ask, 'Danielle, how was your day?' Even if her verdict is 'Nothing' or ''S boring', she should have a chance to get your full attention. They will eventually learn to take turns.
- Children need personal space in the literal sense too, but twins rarely get it. If they still share a bedroom, perhaps each could have his own desk or bookshelf.
- Help each child make his own friends. There may be difficulties to begin with, especially if neither has made

many friends before, or one of them receives more invitations than the other.

- Make a special time to read each child's end-of-term report, if necessary using a kitchen timer to show them you're being scrupulously fair.
- Make sure you congratulate each child on his achievements. Some parents (and teachers) go out of their way not to congratulate a twin who has succeeded well at something, for fear of upsetting the other one. While it is true that the twin who has not done as well as his brother may take it badly, it makes no sense to punish, in effect, the one who comes first by withholding your praise. Like any child, he needs to have a bit of a fuss made over him. This can be quite a tightrope to tread, but would anything else be fair?

· *Dealings with Teachers* ·

- Don't assume that school life simply mirrors what happens at home. Sometimes twins fight at home but not at school, and vice versa. As one seven-year-old told his mum: 'I've been good all day. I can't be good all the time.'
- Make yourself accessible to staff, ready to talk through any niggles as they arise, before they become major worries. Teachers appreciate this and you will get on better as a result.
- Always mention any medical problems or domestic difficulties that may affect your children's behaviour or performance at school.
- Don't forget to ask the teacher if she ever gets your children muddled (very important if they are in the same class). You might be surprised how often teachers confuse identicals – and even non-identicals of the same sex. There may be ways you can help her distinguish them.
- Find out what is happening in class. Are your children in

separate groups? Does each approach the teacher for help? If so, is it for himself or for his sibling? Is each child treated on his own merits? You may be surprised to find out that some teachers will hold back one child (with spellings, times tables, reading or whatever) if his twin is not ready yet.

- What happens at playtime? Do your children just play together or do they mix well with others?

- Liaise with the teacher over sensible homework arrangements. You probably won't be able to help quite as much with your children's homework if you have twins – still less with triplets or quads. If each has to read to you in the evening, it makes more sense for your twins to have different books. Find out too about such things as project work. Your children may fight over who takes out which library book on the Vikings, for instance. Make sure that your children aren't being given identical homework assignments simply because they are twins, while everyone else in the class does something different (this has been known to happen).

- On school outings, same-sex multiples probably ought to be in separate groups, on grounds of safety if nothing else.

- Arrange separate appointments on parents' evenings for each child: perhaps some other parents could go in between your two appointments, just to keep the boundaries clear.

- Don't compare your children. Even for determined parents, this is surprisingly hard to avoid, but each child has to be considered – and encouraged – in his own right.

Treating multiples as individuals is as important at school as it is anywhere else, but of course they are still twins, no matter how different or alike they may be. Twinship creates a special bond which one should neither ignore nor try to break forcibly. And why shouldn't your children enjoy the fact that twinship is special?

Chapter Thirteen

SECONDARY SCHOOL

Jonathan nicked my new shin-pads and he lost one of them. Now I've got a lunch-time detention for not having my kit.[1]

Whatever choices you made about primary schooling, fresh decisions have to be made about secondary education, and here a whole new set of circumstances needs to be considered – all at the awkward age when your offspring are turning into teenagers.

Secondary school calls for new approaches to classwork and home learning. Your children will have many more exams, and lots of coursework. Becoming organised and self-reliant is now a must.

As well as providing an education, secondary schools offer more of an opportunity for twins to become independent, while still enjoying the pleasures that their special bond brings.

You could just send them both to the nearest secondary school and be done with it. After all, isn't that where everyone in your road goes? This may be the right decision, but you need to explore all the options first, and there are now more of them.

· *Same School* ·

The same school is the logical choice for many multiples, especially if they have similar interests and abilities.

[1] The language has been toned down to avoid offending readers.

Adolescents need personal space – and twins need it more than most – but secondary schools, which are often much bigger than primary schools, may provide it without your making difficult (and possibly divisive) arrangements involving different schools.

Same school, same class

If a school has only one class per year group, there may be no choice, though this is unusual. Where the school is big enough to have two or more parallel classes, your twins may well end up in the same one if you don't ask, purely on the basis of their date of birth or the place of their surname in the alphabet! This may not be what you and they had in mind.

Being in the same class is not usually the ideal option at secondary level, especially now that there are more and more exams and increasing social pressures.

Adolescents are more touchy and in greater need of privacy than younger children, and thrive better if they have space. This applies especially to those same-sex pairs where there are marked physical or intellectual differences between them.

Nothing is ever totally black and white, however, and the same class may well work if your children function independently and are of similar ability. Bear in mind, though, that only one of them will be able to come top (or bottom, for that matter) and this can be a big issue at a sensitive age.

Same school, separate classes

Many secondary schools have parallel intakes and two or more classes all the way through. Moreover, your children's existing friends from primary school will probably be distributed more or less equally into the different classes, which could ease the separation of your twins from each other.

My identical boys started at the local comprehensive two years ago and we have no regrets so far. It is a huge school with plenty going on, and both Richard and Magnus have plenty of scope. They've made friends there – in fact, they each had people they knew from primary school in their class when they started. In their lunch break they each pursue activities. Richard does basketball and Magnus is into chess.

Bear in mind, though, that even in separate classes your twins may still be together for some subjects and will probably mix in the playground and the canteen, and for sports and some extra-curricular activities. With same-sex twins there's still potential for teachers to get confused, especially as there's usually a uniform. Pupils try to customise their uniform whenever they can get away with it, but given teenage tribalism they still end up the same as their peers. At the time of writing, that means all the boys have a spike of gelled hair and shirts that hang out, while the girls all hitch up their skirts as much as possible and wear their school ties very short.

In many schools there are several sets for each subject. Sometimes pupils are streamed according to ability. Whether your multiples are in the same set or not, there can be problems. It all depends on your twins. A parent's sensitive handling can help, but sometimes it's better for them to go to entirely different schools.

· *Separate Schools* ·

This can work better than many parents imagine at first. You needn't usually worry about the school run since kids often take themselves to secondary school, depending on local transport. Some evenings they may still need a chauffeur service, though, if one or other stays late for an after-school activity.

Transport can prove expensive if one school is out of your immediate area. In these cases free or reduced-fare travel may not be available. You also need to think about different sports days, prize days and so on.

Separate schools can work particularly well for boy-girl pairs, who often drift apart around puberty. Another important factor is that girls tend to mature (in all senses of the word) much earlier than boys. A teenaged girl usually performs better at school than her male twin. There are still many single-sex schools, both within and outside the state system, and on the whole if there is one for girls in your area, there is often one of a similar standard and ethos for boys nearby too.

Alexis goes to the girls' grammar school while Jasper goes to the boys' one, which is pretty much equivalent in terms of standards and is half a mile away from the girls' school. It is ideal for them (and me) because they come home on the same bus. The only bone of contention is that by the time the bus gets to Jasper's school, all the seats are taken by the girls.

For multiples of very different ability, and perhaps also for those of very similar appearance, separate schools with their different emphasis can help each child fulfil his potential and blossom without the constraint of his twin.

· *Selective Schools* ·

In some schools, admission depends on a child's performance in a test or series of tests, and often interviews as well. In the case of selective schools, especially independent schools, it is worth asking about the policy on siblings. Most independent schools do not automatically give any preference to siblings. However, at the moment some private schools are seeing a fall in the number of applicants, so they're prepared to be more flexible. There may therefore be some leeway here if your children aren't strictly speaking of the same standard but you think it would be a good idea for them to attend the same selective school. Of course you need to know it's what your twins would like too.

The situation is not uniform across the state sector either. A few local authorities won't separate twins into different schools, even when their scores at 12 plus are very different. Other local authorities do the opposite, separating twins when one has reached the required score to get into the selective school and the other has narrowly missed it.

If your twins perform differently and you want them both to go to the same school, you must decide first whether this would be in the best interests of each child as well as being more convenient for you. Naturally, academic results are important, but they are hardly ever the only factor in choosing schools. A school's approach and ethos come into the decision, as do sports facilities and extra-curricular offerings. If you believe there are good reasons for your twins to be together (or apart) despite their exam results, say so. You can also ask Tamba for support in this. Remember that the people you deal with at the education department or even in the individual schools may not have had many direct dealings with multiples – and they certainly won't know your children as well as you do.

· *Choosing Secondary Schools* ·

Few areas are so isolated as to offer no alternatives, and you will need to evaluate several factors in choosing schools.

1 The school itself

There are many different types of school – a huge topic which is outside the scope of this book – but how does one make a choice? How, for that matter, do you reach any decision regarding your children's future? Start by going to open evenings – with your children – and see what you think. Ask the staff how twins are dealt with. Soak up the atmosphere of the school. Do you and your children like it? If you disagree, why is this?

You can also ask other parents in your area about local schools. However, beware of the local grapevine. There's gossip about every school and it's sometimes useless, especially if it is years out of date.

Scan league tables of exam results if you feel so inclined, although even enthusiasts of league tables agree that they do not give the whole picture. As an obvious example, schools with no sixth form will have no scores for A level. However, the main drawback of the tables is undoubtedly that they do not take into account the ability of the pupils admitted, so they do not (yet) reflect the 'value-added' factor.

2   The logistics

Here's where you need to juggle all the practical considerations, such as distance, travel time and perhaps finances. You might, for example, have considered private education, but it can be difficult scraping together two lots of school fees. In this case, investigate bursaries or scholarships (though these last rarely cover more than a fraction of the fees these days). There's also the cost of school trips, sports equipment and extra-curricular activities, which can make it all add up. And school fees do rise. It could be damaging to have to move your children from one school to another at a sensitive time in their education.

3   The children

It is hard always to do the best thing for your children, especially when there are two or more of the same age, but that of course is your mission. If your twins have been together throughout primary school, you may not have a clear picture of how each functions independently. For each child, think carefully about his:

- academic ability
- motivation
- learning style
- interests
- independence from his twin
- social maturity
- need for privacy (often very great in multiples)
- any learning difficulties or special needs
- similarity in appearance to his twin.

Perhaps it is wrong to judge by physical appearance, but it is a fact that people do. It can also affect behaviour. It certainly alters the way outsiders relate to them.

On the whole, MZ (monozygotic or identical) twins are closer than DZ (dizygotic or non-identical) same-sex twins. The relationship between them may be uneven, with one being dominant and the other submissive.

Psychologist Nancy Segal's research has found all twins to be more competitive than co-operative, though MZ twins are less competitive than the DZ twins. Your own research, based on a much smaller sample, may of course suggest otherwise!

Work from educationalist Britta Akerman in Sweden found that teenaged MZ twins tend to be less creative than DZ pairs. But boys in boy-girl pairs are more creative than those in same-sex pairs. She also believes that DZ girls are more confident than MZ girls.

All this may have a bearing on your own children's aptitudes and performance at school.

Your twins should have some say in the matter of their education. They are after all experts at being twins.

Personally I don't think children should have the privilege – or the burden – of making the final decision as to which school they go to, but their views and wishes do matter, and it's important for them to know that they're taken seriously. So find out what they think. Are they keen to be apart (or together)? What do they think of the particular schools you're considering? Where are their friends going to be? Do they have any thoughts about the future? Try to talk to each alone.

One large school with six parallel classes was going to allocate one of two identical 11-year-olds to a class where both had friends from primary school, while his twin would have been in a class where he knew nobody. A word in the headteacher's ear soon changed things. Without too much difficulty, each twin was placed in a class where he knew four or five of his peers.

· *Important Issues at Secondary School* ·

Relatively little research has been done on multiples at secondary school, but according to many twins, parents and teachers, some issues make a regular appearance.

Identity

In school uniform, identical twins may resemble each other so closely that teachers have a great deal of trouble telling them apart. There may be a few centimetres' difference in height, or one may have more freckles, but this is of no use when only one twin is present! If people have to ask who the child is before they are sure, so that every conversation starts with an insensitive: 'Which one are you?' then obviously relationships can suffer.

By the time multiples get to secondary school, it is

important for each to function independently and have a strong sense of their own identity. Most do. However, the security and comfort of being a twin has a particular appeal, especially to a child who is shy, retiring or a little less able. This occasionally creates problems. In some pairs, one twin may continue to make the executive decisions while the other hangs back uncertainly. Moving on to secondary school means becoming a little fish in a bigger pond, and this can accentuate or alter the balance of the relationship between the twins.

Some twins like to show off their twinship as something that makes them special. If they are in different schools, they lose this badge. On the other hand, your children may not particularly like being twins. At secondary school, some twins have been known to conceal their twinship, perhaps in an attempt to break free. Two non-identical boys who went to different schools did this very effectively for nearly two years, without either mentioning to anyone that he had a brother, let alone a twin.

Privacy

This is an issue throughout childhood and the teen years, but it has particular relevance to secondary school. If your twins are at the same school, albeit in separate classes, you may find that one child tells you all about her twin: 'Natalie had to go and see Mrs Worthington again'; 'Natalie fancies Roderick' and so on. Of course, not all twins tell tales on each other, but when they do, you can bet Natalie will get fed up with it. And she will retaliate as soon as she gets a chance.

Privacy over school life is essential – no child has a right to know his twin's results and still less to blurt them out as soon as he gets halfway through the front door. Whether the news is good or less good, each child should have his moment to share it with his parents in private. Whether multiples should see each other's reports varies from family to family. Obviously the children should only do so if they agree, a point which also applies to exam results.

> *Alex had let Kim hear the marks on his end-of-year report, but Kim wasn't reciprocating because his own report, although very good, wasn't quite as glowing. Both boys ended up hopping mad. Instead of congratulating each of them, the evening was eaten up in trying to placate them.*

Each child also needs a private place to work, and to do nothing if he chooses, away from the prying eyes of a sibling with Scotland Yard tendencies. Separate bedrooms are ideal, but not every family can provide that luxury. Some sort of partition across a bedroom can work, though it has occasionally been known for a dividing curtain to get pulled down in a fit of teen pique.

Behaviour

Boisterous children settle down eventually, but naughtiness can persist into secondary school, and 'twin-power' may make it hard to handle. Sometimes one twin behaves badly and the other follows suit to avoid feeling left out. The end result is much the same and both end up in trouble. Again, the balance may change, and you may find that the follower becomes the leader, or that the one who is usually reserved becomes far less quiet.

Sometimes clowning around and other disruptive behaviour in class only surfaces when the twins come together for certain lessons after they have become used to being taught separately for a year or more. It may be a knee-jerk response to the chemistry of being together again, but occasionally it is a deliberate ploy to get attention from teacher or classmates.

Disruptive behaviour can also be due to inattention and

lack of concentration. Attention deficit disorder, or ADHD, is more common in twins, especially boys (see Appendix, page 363). It's now known that it can persist into adolescence and even adulthood, and if one of your children has it, there may be important consequences for behaviour and learning. It's hard to be organised if you can't follow through complex instructions like 'Brush your teeth, clean your shoes, and make sure you've got your chemistry homework.'

Homework

Compared with primary school, different skills are needed now. Pupils need to be organised for different lessons in different classrooms, and have to motivate themselves and manage their time. Even when they are in different classes or at different schools, twins may well have similar homework assignments because of the National Curriculum. It's tempting to let them help each other, but this can be counter-productive. Each must learn to work independently.

There is scope for some compromise in certain areas, for instance sharing books for a project. Oddly enough, though, this is when some multiples argue fiercely.

One of them got three library books on forestry and his brother only found one. Each guarded his jealously and we were treated to tantrums the like of which we hadn't seen for years.

However, they can work well together. Several mothers have told me that their twins help each other out. Twin-power can be a good thing when practising French conversation, or testing each other, but there is a danger here too, according to one mother (who is also a teacher):

It's very tempting just to let them get on with it, but I know that, although they have each other, parents still need to be involved with schoolwork and show an interest.

Problems can arise when one of the twins gets more homework than the other, perhaps because of different teaching styles. Officially there may be three homework subjects a night, but it doesn't always work out that evenly. The one with more work on any one evening is likely to think it's grossly unfair and may fail to complete it, or else rush through it so he can join his twin slumped in front of the telly.

Different abilities

As at primary school, a disparity in ability can cause intense jealousy between twins, as well as heartache for parents. Most of us, consciously or not, still expect twins to be just the same. When there are only tiny differences, we parents can get hung up about them. At any one point, you probably consider one of your twins 'better' at school. The danger is that the 'worse' one may stop trying.

The drawbacks of comparing multiples have already cropped up in Chapters 9 and 12. This can continue to cause problems at secondary school, but now there's a new slant on issues thanks to puberty – especially when twins go through it at different times (see Chapter 14).

We are not all the same, but everyone has some talent. In the case of a less able child, you have to uncover it so that he can channel his energy and enthusiasm. Multiples can change in their relative abilities around now, and the twin who did well before may trail behind now. Both twins need to maintain self-respect.

There are times when different aptitudes can hurt:

Matthew got picked for the school football team and Andrew didn't, even though he thought he was the better player. He obviously wasn't, and he was gutted. But he got over it eventually and he now plays hockey.

Sports and music are obvious outlets, but not the only ones. In one pair of non-identical boys, one brother was both more able and much more athletic. His twin did not appear to be good at anything until he discovered sleight of hand. Now his small build and newly found capacity for telling jokes make him a popular amateur magician who specialises in entertaining at younger children's parties (earning him far more than his twin gets from a distinctly unglamorous paper round).

Exams

Revising for and sitting exams is very stressful for any child. With twins, a double dose of 'exam crisis' can seriously affect the whole family. And then there are the results. You must of course congratulate whoever does well, even if this seems unfair because one twin gets most of the praise. It would be less fair to treat them equally if their efforts were unequal. After all, you don't want to heap praise on the one who did much less work.

For those children who feel their results must match their twin's, the pressure to achieve may be enormous. If they are of different aptitudes it may be impossible. GCSEs and A levels create particularly trying times. They should have got over such feelings by the time they get to GCSEs, and most have. But with some twins, even minor differences in performance can lead to envy, sulking or guilt.

One girl learned her stunning A level results from the notice-board, but her heart sank because she was worried about her twin sister's marks. She felt guilty since she knew her sister couldn't have done as brilliantly.

For this reason, some twins try hard not to do too well. There may also be an element of inverted snobbery: teenage boys in particular consider it uncool to succeed academically.

Parents and grandparents sometimes offer rewards for

good results, dangling a carrot for certain grades in GCSEs or A levels. What if only one of your multiples reaches the required level? And can you afford it if all of them surpass expectations? Think very hard before signing up to offers like these.

Though they may seem interminable, exams do eventually end. As one parent says, 'Results arrive, for better or for worse. You live through it, and life moves on.'

Teachers' attitudes

As a parent, one expects teachers to be experts in all aspects of education, but this is not always the case. Like all professionals – lawyers, doctors, and so on – teachers have their own interests and they are not all equally gifted in every subject or with every pupil. The reality is that not every single teacher has the unbiased professional approach you want to see.

Many teachers, remember, have had little or no training in the issues facing multiples at school. As at primary level, parents have to be prepared to co-operate closely and to point teachers in the right direction, preferably gently and tactfully (you catch more bears with honey). It is harder keeping in touch with teachers when your children are at secondary school, but you can try. Tamba provides useful study days and other resources for teachers, and you can also point schools in the direction of the website *www.twinsandmultiples.org*.

· *Choices for the Future* ·

There are no hard-and-fast rules for parents. It would be easier if your twins went their separate ways during and after school and made different career choices. Then nobody would judge their performance relative to each other.

It came as a shock to me when we were posted abroad to find that only one of our 16-year-old sons was planning on joining us. His brother wanted to go to boarding school back home and concentrate on his music. I don't think I was prepared for such a sudden and total separation, but if I'm honest I've always known they had different inclinations. And I'm proud that Mark felt able to make that decision.

However, many twins do choose the same subjects for their GCSEs and A levels. Some are genuinely interested in the same things. For example, one twin, now in middle age, lectures in Japanese at Oxford while his identical twin is professor of Chinese at Cambridge. Both also do work on eastern religions. After all, many non-twin siblings share interests too and there is no shortage of children who follow in a parent's footsteps.

While helping each of your offspring to be individuals, it is important not to separate them forcibly. Different options for GCSE and A level may lead to misery if chosen for the wrong reasons. In Britain, the trend is still to specialise in just a few subjects at AS and A level, and this forces young people to make tough decisions at an early age.

As for any youngster, it is essential for twins to make choices that are appropriate for them rather than because they suit someone else's agenda. There is also an element of chance and timing in selecting colleges and universities; sometimes it just depends on who got their form in first.

So if your children seem to want the same career, instead of trying to get them to change their minds, aim to find out why. Have they explored all their options? Are their interests genuinely similar? Or are they afraid of leading adult lives which are too separate? If they have had good opportunities so far, this is unlikely to be the case. However, separate colleges or universities can be very traumatic if your twins have never been apart before.

Sometimes multiples leave school at different times. There's little a parent can do, but you should discuss all the implications with your youngster and tell him (preferably calmly) what your opinion is. Young adults should be treated as adults, but that doesn't stop you from giving your views. It also shows your offspring that you do care.

If your twins choose widely divergent paths, is this because they are twins and feel the need to be different? You need to look at this too.

Twins needn't necessarily drift away from each other because they attend different colleges or pursue different vocations. Even multiples at very distant universities may continually phone each other and spend more spare time and holidays together than they do with their parents. Don't worry. They'll soon be home with their dirty washing.

· *What Can Parents Do?* ·

Although you can't change your twins fundamentally, even if you want to, you can still usefully apply some of the ideas from the previous chapter. You may not have to do much at all: by this stage, many twins are well adjusted to functioning independently and sail through secondary school with no more hiccups than anyone else. As some parents find, even identical twins tend to diverge more and more in the teen years and end up delightfully different. All you have to do is take the credit.

If you haven't already, try to:

- provide as much privacy as possible for each child
- provide as much space as possible (own desk, own room or whatever you can manage)

- encourage them not to compete for marks, friends, etc.
- treat them as individuals – no calling out for 'the Twinnies' when one of them is wanted on the phone
- be sympathetic and supportive: let each of them tell you how she feels
- find something each is good at, but don't force them into separate choices just for the sake of it – multiples, especially identicals, may have the same interests
- go easy on unimportant issues: some things which make you see red now may not matter a bit in a year from now
- at all costs, avoid making comparisons. Don't ever try to discipline one twin by complaining that his brother is always so much better behaved!
- agree with them when they complain that life's unfair – it is, and it's a tough lesson to learn.

· *Parents' Evenings* ·

These can be something of an endurance test for parents of multiples; even those who only have singletons find it hard to whizz round trying to see all the teachers in one evening and remember what was said. Here are some suggestions from parents of twins about making it work:

- Take a notebook and pencil. You may just about remember what six different teachers said about one child (and the points you want to raise), but with twins or more you will definitely need something to jog your memory.
- If you have a partner, perhaps he could see one child's teachers while you deal with those of the other twin.
- If you cannot see all the staff on parents' evening, concentrate on meeting the teachers who seem most vital for each child. You could explain your predicament to the

school in advance and ask their advice as to whom you really must see.

- Go on two separate evenings if you can, or arrange to see some teachers at another time, perhaps just before or after classes one schoolday.
- If you can't do this, use the phone. Many teachers are happy to let you know when they can take calls. Sometimes email is good too.
- Even if your children have the same teachers, always stick to discussing one child at a time, as at primary school.
- There may be times when the twinship is an issue. If so, make opportunities to keep teachers up to date with what's happening, and be prepared to discuss both children together on these occasions.

Chapter Fourteen

ADOLESCENCE AND THE TEEN YEARS

Parents would die if they knew what we were really like.

No, that wasn't from a present-day teenager, but attributed to poet Rupert Brooke nearly a hundred years ago, which shows that there's nothing all that new about parent–adolescent conflicts.

Adolesco is Latin for 'I grow up'. Adolescence, the process of becoming an adult, can put years on the parents too. When my own twins reached their first birthday, I could finally foresee an end to the round-the-clock demands of babycare and I recall confidently telling a friend that with twins the first year was the worst. Being the father of twins himself, he disagreed. 'With twins,' he replied, 'the first 20 years are the worst.'

It was said in jest, but contains a grain of truth. For many parents of twins, adolescence is a time when their children grow further apart and rebel against the twinship. Twins don't necessarily have a stormier adolescence, but different issues can arise. The adolescent twin is faced not just with breaking away from parental control but also with separating from his co-twin. All the evidence suggests that the earlier in life this process starts, and the more used each child is to being treated as an individual in his own right, the easier adolescence is. But, however exemplary your raising of your twins has been so far, you cannot rely on having an easy ride in the teen years. In fact, you can't count on anything much during these sometimes painful years.

There are good reasons for the turmoils of adolescence and puberty. First, though, they're two different stages that overlap. Puberty is the time when a human acquires the ability to reproduce. This typically happens over a period of two to three years, beginning between the ages of 10 to 14 in boys and nine to 13 in girls. Adolescence is a more extended stage. Encompassing puberty, it's the final phase of physical and emotional maturation that turns a child into an adult.

· *What is Happening* ·

There's a lot going on. Puberty itself involves a complex cauldron of hormones bubbling away. In both sexes it starts with a rise in secretion of the hormone GnRH (short for gonadotrophin releasing hormone) from the hypothalamus, a small but significant part of the brain. The main effect of GnRH is to make the anterior pituitary gland, again hidden deep inside the brain, release LH (luteinising hormone) and FSH (follicle-stimulating hormone). From early puberty, the pituitary produces LH in pulses, especially at night, until eventually LH levels are steady at a new high level as in adults. These hormones are exactly the same in both girls and boys, but their effects differ. In boys, the new hormonal environment makes the testicles secrete testosterone and grow. In girls, the ovaries respond by producing oestrogen and progesterone. But during puberty there's also a slight rise in testosterone in girls and oestrogen in boys. In a nutshell, that's why teenaged girls can get spots and oily skin too, and why 14-year-old boys can get unwelcome breast tenderness and enlargement.

What makes GnRH rise in the first place? For the moment that's a mystery, though size seems to matter. The onset of puberty is linked with reaching a critical body weight – around 47 kg (7½ stone) for girls and 55 kg (8½ stone) for boys. This partly explains why twins don't always go through puberty at the same time.

The other main feature of puberty is increase in height, thanks to growth hormone (GH) from the pituitary. Girls start their growth spurt at about 10 or 11, and grow around 25 cm (10 inches). Boys grow about 28 cm (11 inches), but don't start shooting upwards until some two years later, when they've become taller. This accounts for the average height difference of 13 cm (5 inches) between adult men and women. Research shows that most twins reach their target grown-up height, though some are slightly underweight compared with singletons. MZ (monozygotic or identical) twins tend to grow in a similar style to each other, DZ (dizygotic or non-identical) twins less so.

Growth hormone makes a youngster grow by promoting protein manufacture – and that means teens need to eat. No wonder they tend to raid the kitchen, often at very anti-social times, as judged by their parents. They also need to sleep, hence the tendency to lie in late.

This soup of hormones has effects other than on growth and sex organs. Sweating is linked with testosterone, so it tends to be worse in boys, and poses another social handicap for the gawky adolescent. Skin problems, again mostly due to testosterone, plague some three-quarters of all teenagers.

Hormones also affect behaviour and thought. It's the male hormone testosterone that increases sex drive in both girls and boys, which is one reason why adolescents have sex on the brain. Oestrogen and progesterone probably also affect sexual behaviour, though in a less obvious way. Clearly there are lots of social and cultural influences at work too.

Oestrogen and progesterone almost certainly cause moodiness, while testosterone fuels aggression. Shyness and embarrassment may be due to hormones, and so too may symptoms like depression. It's said that around 10 per cent of teenagers are depressed. The figure is no higher in twins, and studies suggest they are not often distressed at the same time.

There's some suggestion that genes can get switched on at puberty so that new characteristics emerge. This may also mean that the balance of power between your twins changes, and they may become more or less alike.

· *What Adolescence is Like* ·

There may be no such thing as growing pains, but, as the eminent paediatrician John Apley put it, 'Physical growth does not hurt, though emotional growth can hurt like hell!' If you can't remember your own teenage years in all their awfulness, try to imagine what it must be like to go through all that physical and mental upheaval at a time when there are mounting educational and social pressures.

Of course, adolescents can be incredibly selfish. You the parent may be lying ill in bed, or working hard at your high-powered job, but you'll be expected to jump to attention whenever one of your teens needs a cheque for £50 for her imminent school trip, her favourite blouse washed and ready to wear now, or a lift to a mate's house.

When she's thwarted, as for example when you need the phone for a change, she may have tantrums. You'll also find that teenagers don't like being told what to do. The more you remind them to do something, the less likely it is to get done (unless you do it yourself).

Where else do you see such behaviour? In toddlerhood, that's where. Teenagers and their quest for independence have much in common with two-year-olds. I like to think of adolescence as the deluxe version of toddlerhood, with a sexual element thrown in for good measure. One other important distinction: your children are now way too big to pick up and plonk in a corner.

At this point you may be forgiven for looking back wistfully on those earlier years, when your twins were so cute and so much more manageable. This doesn't always make the adolescent's lot any easier.

I still think of my twins, now 16, as my babies. Sometimes I'll even call them 'Baby'. I know I shouldn't, but somehow it just slips out.

Teenagers need approval, but as a parent beware of how you give it. The average teenager doesn't want his mother to think he looks 'sweet' or 'very smart, dear' – he'd much rather look like his peers, in other words like some unspeakable Goth, quite possibly complete with metalwork.

As idealists, adolescents often get despondent about the future. True depression does occur in this age group, but many more youngsters are simply worried about life choices. It's probably raging hormones that make teenagers so intense, reacting to even minor irritants. Whatever the reason, the most trivial things can end up getting on their nerves – yours too, of course.

They also tend to be highly critical of others and of the adult world at large. Moods can change, though, from one minute to the next. To a parent, the see-saws in ideas and emotions can seem violent.

Teenagers tend to be very territorial and you may hear each of your twins talking much more about 'my room', 'my CDs' or whatever. Nonetheless, they're still likely to borrow your things and fail to return them.

Adolescence comes at a time when they are bombarded from all sides by images and messages that suggest they should be good-looking, super-cool, slim and so on. No wonder a single spot can be a disaster of national significance.

For the parent, adolescence may come at a time when many other things are going on. If your twins were born

when you were 35, which is not unusual, during most of their
teen years you will be in your fifties, and possibly coping with
the difficulties of the menopause, redundancy or forthcoming
retirement. Divorce rates are continuing to rise, so you may
be caring for teenaged twins on your own, with all the
practical and emotional burdens that single parenthood
entails. Caring for elderly relatives may also consume your
time and energies. Where will you find a few moments for
yourself in all this?

· *Some Practical Problems of* · *Teenaged Twins*

Puberty

Twins (and triplets) often mature at different times. It is
normal for girls to go through puberty two years ahead of
boys. This is often when the girl of a mixed-sex pair will be
more mature in both looks and attitude, as well as taller than
her twin because she has already had her adolescent growth
spurt and he has not.

One lad developed a cute strategy for dealing with this:

*We're not twins. She's two years older than me, but we're in the
same class because she's so thick.*

Same-sex pairs, and even identical twins, can also go through
puberty at different times, however, as paediatrician Dr John
Buckler confirms. There may be an interval of six months or
a year before they both reach the same physical stage. This
has many implications:

● If twins appear to be of different ages, the outward signs of
  twinship are in effect lost.

- The effect of looking more mature is that people expect you to behave in a more adult way.
- Those who mature later (especially boys) seem to suffer more crises of confidence.
- Puberty makes one highly sensitive about one's body. Pubertal twins desperately need privacy, all the more so if they're at different stages of physical development.
- An adolescent twin can become acutely aware of being less attractive (or less well endowed) than his or her same-sex twin.

Identity

Self-esteem depends crucially on identity – as the cliché goes, every adolescent tries to find himself. This can be a time of deep ambiguity of feelings. On the one hand, twins often value the special bond they have, but on the other they may rebel against it.

Even if they have been happy looking alike, in adolescence twins often consider it important to appear different. That's why you can get some same-sex (even identical) twins choosing to dress in completely contrasting styles. Sometimes they succeed, sometimes they don't:

> *My daughters think they're dressing differently, but they're both in black all the time and it may as well be a uniform.*

In an attempt to look dissimilar, two identical girls of 17 each went to the hairdresser's separately and asked for their lovely long hair to be cut. Each just asked for 'a style that'll suit me'. They both emerged with exactly the same bob.

Independence

In a same-sex pair, the dominant twin may continue to make

all the decisions and take the lead. The dominant one is often (though not necessarily) the one who is more advanced physically.

Dominance may change in adolescence. Sometimes one wants to break free, while the other doesn't – a situation which can be as painful as the break-up of any relationship. It is often the less dominant teenager who sees the light and wants to leave his twin's shadow. Meanwhile, the so-called dominant partner may begin to feel insecure without the constant quiet presence of his twin.

In girl-boy pairs, the boy may become protective of his sister, acting as her chaperon and/or defender of her morals. She may resent it. On the other hand, her brother's presence can have advantages, especially if you allow her to stay out later as a result.

> *My brother was often at the same parties and our parents thought that was great. I know they didn't worry at all because we were together. But then, they didn't know that he was legless most of the time.*

Whether they're the same sex or not, allowing twins to go out together can be convenient – surely there's safety in numbers? This is not always best for their individual development and may inhibit one or both. One of a set of identical girls was always the leader, going around with a wild crowd who often got into trouble. Not wishing to be left behind, her far more introverted sister just tagged along, unhappy to be with them, yet unhappy on her own.

Friendships

Several people, including family therapist Audrey Sandbank, have pointed out that twins often start dating later than singletons: no bad thing, you may think, since kids seem to grow up so soon these days. This is probably a reflection of the fact that twins have each other for company and hence less immediate need of others. But the time will come.

It can be awkward for them to make friends of either sex. Many parents of teenaged twins comment that, although their children have lots of friends, they do not have one or two very close ones. Perhaps outsiders are reluctant to intrude on the special relationship twins often have. When one of them does have a best friend, intense jealousy can result, with the other twin feeling left out or even trying to share the friend.

· *Single-parent Issues* ·

It is demanding enough for two parents to deal with the ups and downs of one teenager, so how does one adult alone cope with two or more adolescents?

Those who head single-parent families may find it very tough bringing up children without a resident role model of the opposite gender. There can be many other practical and financial problems when you are on your own: single parents may be lonely, isolated socially and in reduced circumstances.

It is hard for a lone parent to have the conviction to support his or her own point of view without the reinforcement and feedback of a partner. In the case of twins, it can be particularly difficult to be consistent and firm when faced with an onslaught of demands from more than one awkward adolescent. No wonder there are times when it is much easier just to give in and say 'yes' rather than 'no' to two or more stroppy teenagers.

On the other hand, the juggling act that single parents have to perfect has its rewards. Consistency in handling your children is less of a problem – after all, there is no one to undermine you or persuade you to overturn your decisions!

Children of lone parents, far from running wild, are often quite mature in their emotions, very supportive of their parent and able to show insight and understanding.

Everyone wants a piece of you, Mum.

Single-parent households are frequently noted for the closeness of the parent–child relationship, and families of twins are no exception. As a single parent comes through this difficult time, he or she may often feel a fantastic amount of pride in the twins, and quite right too. But the flip side is that it can be especially painful to let the youngsters go, particularly if they both leave home at the same time.

Tamba's One-Parent Families Group offers information and support from other members.

· *What Can Parents Do to Help* · *Adolescents?*

All youngsters are different, and to some extent adolescence is uncharted territory, but there are ways of making things easier:

- Make sure there are behavioural boundaries, but avoid being critical. Nobody, least of all a teenager, functions well against a constant soundtrack of criticism. As for anger, it's best to save it for something illegal, immoral or genuinely outrageous. *You* decide if it matters what their bedrooms look like.
- Use appropriate ways to show you love them. Although they are growing up, they still need parental love and even the odd hug.
- Avoid labelling your twins. In your head you may have the

same old labels for them, but they're likely to be out of date.

- Give each twin as much privacy as you can provide. This includes emotional privacy, the security of knowing he can be listened to without his twin being there or hearing all about it later. Watch out for teenagers who eavesdrop.
- Don't take advantage of the twin relationship. For many years, your children may have understood each other intuitively, but in adolescence and beyond it is important to resist asking one effectively to tell on the other.
- Try not to assume that they will look out for each other's physical or emotional welfare. It is not necessarily a youngster's fault that his twin is upset.
- Allow your twins to work out their own relationship. There are many advantages to having a twin and you can sometimes help by emphasising the positive side of twinship. However, try not to envy them. You won't win anyone over by saying, 'If only I'd had a twin sister at your age I'd have loved it, not whinged about it all the time.'
- Don't assume that your twins still have the same likes and dislikes, or want similar presents at Christmas. Even if they're identical, adolescence is a time when their tastes can diverge dramatically.
- Many twins will want separate birthday parties at this age, on different days, with different guests. On the other hand, many do not mind sharing a birthday, contrary to what many parents may imagine. It is better to ask them than to make assumptions.
- Teenagers' self-esteem can be boosted if they are given more responsibility or a part-time job. Twins may be ready to look after younger siblings – and to baby-sit for other families – at a slightly earlier age than singletons.
- If your children are still angelic, don't be fooled into thinking that they'll always be the heavenly twins. Their adolescent rebellion may just come a little later than it does for singletons.

- Finally, hang on to your sense of humour. Seeing the funny side can help get everyone through adolescent traumas, and you may need this more than most, especially if your twins both play drums or electric guitar. Or when they both want lifts simultaneously. Or cars . . .

Once they have grown up, you will no doubt feel a deep sense of achievement. Meanwhile, I strongly recommend Richard Carlson's book *Don't Sweat the Small Stuff . . . and it's all Small Stuff*. It's not specifically about parenting, but it's very apt, not least its subtitle: *Simple Ways to Keep the Little Things from Overtaking Your Life*.

Chapter Fifteen

SPECIAL SITUATIONS, SPECIAL NEEDS

My triplet girls were born at 27 weeks and were in Special Care for over three months each. Our older daughter Katie was three years old at the time, and we included her in everything. She took it all on board without making a fuss – her dolls often had cardiac arrests, and she'd put them on ventilators made of Duplo bricks. People were horrified, but it was her way of coping. Now it is nine years on. The younger three all have special needs but all four girls are well adjusted and play nicely together. Even in the bleakest days, when I was told one or more would die, I was hopeful and kept hanging on. Now I count myself lucky.

Having twins is generally a joyful business. Many a mother has jollied herself along through trying times with her multiples with the thought that she can put up with almost anything as long as the children are healthy.

Sadly, there are circumstances in which one or other twin has some disability or does not survive. This chapter is for these families. Not every special need is covered here, but I hope there will be something to help most parents facing such a situation.

· *Special Needs* ·

Special needs is a term applied to children whose development, communication abilities, learning or behaviour are such that they need special provision to realise their full potential. Although the vast majority of multiple-birth children are completely healthy, the overall rate of special needs is greater in twins and higher multiples than in singletons. The main reasons are:

- prematurity
- poor growth in the womb ('small for dates' infants)
- sometimes, complications of pregnancy (e.g. twin-to-twin transfusion syndrome or pre-eclampsia)
- advances in neonatal care which increase the survival of vulnerable babies who, once upon a time, might not have lived.

A few experts also suggest that the twinning process itself could be a factor implicated in some disabilities in identical (monozygotic or MZ) twins. This is possible, though the theory is still speculative at this point.

Different kinds of special needs

As with any child, the range of conditions that can affect twins is very wide, from trivial to severe and from rare to fairly common. Some are so unusual that they affect only a small number of families in the entire country, but there are many more common problems:

- cerebral palsy (the risk is between three and six times higher in twins and perhaps ten to twenty times higher in triplets)
- various congenital heart defects, such as ventricular or atrial septal defects ('hole in the heart') and transposition of the great vessels
- delayed mental development or learning difficulties.

When one twin is born with a problem, often his twin isn't. Discordance is the medical term for this situation. Its opposite, concordance, means that both twins have the same condition. However, concordant twins aren't necessarily affected to exactly the same degree: one twin can be healthier than the other.

Surprisingly, discordance is usual in otherwise identical twins, especially in congenital heart disease. One theory is that the splitting of the fertilised egg to form each twin may have an effect on midline organs like the heart, gullet, and so on. Perhaps one twin ends up with fewer cells from the splitting.

Effects on the family

Whatever the nature or the underlying cause, disability in a child affects the whole family. With twins, the presence of a healthy child of the same age often means that a problem is picked up sooner. For instance, a delay in one baby in starting to talk or crawl is very obvious when the other one is developing in leaps and bounds.

Clearly, the effects go far deeper. When only one twin has special needs, the presence of the other twin can be a poignant and sometimes painful reminder of what might have been – or, as some parents say, of what should have been.

The parents

Losing the health of your child is a form of bereavement. There may also be grief over the apparent loss of the twin-ship. Many parents comment on how painful it is for them to come across pairs of able-bodied twins, and some go to great lengths to avoid it if they can.

Some mothers feel their loss of status as a parent of twins

very acutely. While a few continue to go to some effort to preserve outward appearances of twin-ness (with identical clothes, for instance), others prefer not to remind themselves or outsiders of the twinship. The comparisons which seem to be an almost inevitable aspect of twinship can be too hard to bear.

The parents of a special needs child may feel intensely guilty or angry. These emotions are perhaps irrational and even unproductive, but understandable none the less. The anger directed at medical professionals can be all the greater when multiples resulted from fertility treatment.

Sometimes parents may find it hard to believe that the remaining healthy twin or triplets are all right. Especially in the early days, the well children are sometimes taken repeatedly to the doctor's, just to make sure. However, this eventually stops – the parents either come to believe that the child is healthy or are simply kept too busy attending to the sick one's needs.

The burden of caring for a less able youngster is obviously far greater when he is one of multiples, because there is already so much to do. When both twin babies are disabled, a mother (and it usually is the mother) may find it impossible to cope. Inevitably, little time is left for the parents to spend with each other. Shortage of time and energy, and often money too, leads to severe restrictions on what a family can do. The logistic problems can result in social isolation. This is hard for any parent, but especially, perhaps, for a mother who has until now had her own career.

Extended family, friends or neighbours may be prepared to help, but special skills are often needed to look after the child, which deters many parents from accepting.

Much of the help given to a family with special needs is aimed at the affected children and their mum. Dads tend to become marginalised, although they have needs as well. Even if he is hesitant to express himself, a father too can feel angry, guilty, cheated or overwhelmed. He may have even more anxieties than his partner.

> *Geoff was always either at the office or helping me out. He is their dad, but he rarely ever got a chance to go to Cormac's school, or see the doctors, to find out how well our son was getting on.*

A father needs to be involved from the early days and to receive support in a form he finds acceptable.

Some parents of disabled twins do, it seems, physically abuse their children, especially if only one twin is disabled. This can only make a difficult situation worse and obviously calls for intervention. Cruelty to children is hard to understand and easy to condemn, but those of us with healthy offspring can barely begin to imagine what the pressures are like.

The special-needs twin

His burdens and limitations are often obvious. In time, he will be able to understand why he does not have the same abilities as his twin, and this needs to be discussed.

People may go out of their way to encourage him. This sometimes means he gets undue praise for his achievements. Many less able-bodied people prefer just to get on with doing the tasks they can manage. This is particularly true of children with cerebral palsy, who are often of normal or even high intelligence, and don't appreciate being patronised.

Being a multiple can have advantages. A more able twin can be a source of companionship, laughter and even motivation. This can help keep the special-needs twin occupied and stimulated.

The healthy twin

Parents of one disabled twin often try hard to be fair to both children. This is especially difficult since time is so short, and whatever they do, it may simply not seem enough. It is inevitable that the healthier of the two will get less attention, but the child may not see it that way. Why should his brother's first syllable or faltering step be so ecstatically acclaimed, while he has been doing far more than this for absolutely ages without a word of praise? He may also have trouble understanding that you tolerate different standards of behaviour from his twin, just because he has special needs.

The healthier twin may indulge in showing off or other forms of attention-seeking, or he may regress until (not surprisingly) his behaviour comes to resemble that of his disabled twin.

Later on, the healthy twin sometimes feels guilty, not simply for his own awkward behaviour but perhaps for his twin's condition, as if he were in some way responsible for it. He may just feel guilty about being the healthy survivor, or he may be under pressure to help care for his twin (though he should never have to).

Some healthy siblings are remarkably well adjusted and take it all in their stride, however:

> *I've done my best to be fair, but I know I haven't always succeeded. Inevitably I spend far more time and effort on Paul, who has needed heart surgery several times. As far as David (the healthy twin) is concerned, he's accepted it and he's been brilliant. But then he's never known any different.*

If one twin is disabled, he is automatically different. It may be an advantage in these circumstances if neither he nor his co-twin thinks of himself as a twin:

> *We never discouraged Robert from thinking of himself as a twin,*

but we never harped on about it either. He just never particularly thought of himself as in any way twinned with his brother, apart from having to share a birthday. They've been different from the word go in all sorts of ways, physically and because of Gavin's gullet problem and his learning difficulties.

In this case, Robert is quite supportive of his less able brother, but mixed feelings are common. Some twins are acutely embarrassed by their twin's special needs. They may prefer to conceal the twinship from their friends.

A few healthy twins learn to grow up fast, becoming mature, sensitive and independent. They should never have to be responsible for the special-needs twin. However, they sometimes take on tasks more suitable for an older child and can become very protective of the less able twin. Again, the difference between the fit child and his special-needs twin is an obvious factor here. Perhaps it is also significant that the healthier twin is often looked after by various friends or relatives, while the less able one gets Mum. Sometimes being, in effect, farmed out results in clinginess, but in other cases the child swiftly learns about separation.

For practical reasons, outings are often restricted. Even with appropriate access, a visit to a museum may be unsuitable for the disabled child. For many years the only outings for the healthy twin may be tedious protracted outpatient visits, tagging along with his sibling.

The healthier child may be desperate to go to Disney World like his school friends, but this may be out of the question for the time being at least. Holidays are often restricted to short breaks nearer home and even then can be anything but restful. One family with special-needs triplets always made sure they chose a campsite near a hospital with an accident and emergency department.

The work of special schools, MBF and Tamba shows that the special needs of the healthy twin are not always recognised, let alone consistently met. To focus on the issues facing the healthy twin, paediatricians Christine Burton and Elizabeth Bryan of the MBF carried out a survey of parents of only one disabled twin.

They found that most parents had little trouble explaining the disability to the healthy sibling, but there were huge difficulties in dealing with it. The overwhelming majority of parents believed that the disability had affected the well child and that he often received less attention, and at times fewer presents too.

The healthy twin sometimes had problems, either behavioural difficulties (feeding, sleeping, tantrums, etc.) or physical ailments like asthma and eczema. Because of the small size of the survey, it is impossible to know whether these are significantly more common in twins with a disabled co-twin, but they might be.

On occasion, friends and professionals who came to the house virtually ignored the healthy one. One or two parents commented that professionals weren't understanding about the significance of the twinship. One paediatrician had apparently told a mother of one twin with cerebral palsy that being a twin 'shouldn't make any difference'.

This survey suggests that some professionals could do better. It also points the way for further work on the long-term effects on a family of having a multiple with special needs.

· *Getting Help* ·

Families with one or more multiples with special needs require information about the disability itself, financial and practical assistance and long-term emotional and social support. Help is at hand from various groups and agencies.

Doctors and other professionals play an obvious role in

assessing and treating special-needs children, and in arranging such things as specialist referrals, physiotherapy, special diets and adaptations to the home. While many GPs and specialists also form the backbone of support for a family, some are not very good at explaining the disability itself – its nature, causes, and long-term outlook.

> *The paediatrician just announced, 'I think one of your twins has got Down's syndrome.' Then he left the room. What did he mean, 'think'? I needed to know. I also needed to know what would become of James and what kind of life he'd have. The staff nurse wasn't encouraging. She told me to expect him to be no more than a vegetable. Fortunately, that's not the case at all. Both he and his twin start at a normal school this year.*

The wide variety of patient groups – from Arthritis Care to the Williams Syndrome Foundation – do an excellent job of providing information in an accessible form. In many cases they also help support the family with a sympathetic ear, a network of local groups and information on the various benefits and allowances they could get.

Support groups play an additional role in raising public and professional awareness and stimulating (and often funding) medical research.

As soon as they can, parents should contact the appropriate support group, but this is only possible if they have a diagnosis. Sometimes there isn't one, or else the child's disorder is so rare that there are only a few sufferers in the entire country. In this case, families are unlikely ever to meet another child with the same disorder. For these, the national charity Contact-a-Family (see Resources, page 373) is an invaluable resource, helping families whose children have a rare or undiagnosed condition.

Tamba's Special Needs Group supports families with one or more multiples who have disabilities. This committed group, run by parents, produces a regular newsletter with advice and views, and creates a contact network for those who want to get in touch with others in a similar situation. Tamba also provides immediate telephone advice via the freephone Twinline (see Resources, page 372). MBF has information for professionals and families about special needs.

Many families with disabled twins benefit from the support of friends, relatives and voluntary workers. One mother tells of her good luck in meeting another family who had twins one year older with the same condition:

> *I knew that whatever difficulties I faced, there was someone else I could talk to who not only knew what it was like, but had lived through exactly that stage already – and survived.*

· *Special Educational Needs* ·

Sometimes one or other school-aged twin has special educational needs. There is quite a lot of relevant legislation, including the Education Act 1993, the Education (Special Needs) (England) Regulations 2001, the Disabilities Discrimination Act 1995 and the Education Act 2002. There is also a Code of Practice which gives guidance to schools, education authorities and others on how best to identify, assess and provide for pupils with special educational needs.

The child's needs could be mild or severe, temporary or permanent, but must be addressed so that the child can benefit as much as possible from education generally and the National Curriculum in particular. The entire process needs partnership between parents and the agencies and professionals involved; an important principle embodied in the code of practice is that the parents' wishes should be taken into account. It does not necessarily follow that their wishes will be granted, however. Parents can appeal to an independent body, the Special Educational Needs tribunal, but the process can take a long time and is sometimes expensive.

For a child with special educational needs, there are several stages of assessment, starting with the point at which concern is raised. The concern might be about anything from poor counting to disruptive behaviour from ADHD (see Appendix, page 363) – and, incidentally, gifted youngsters are also considered to have special educational needs.

In England and Wales, every state school (and a number of independent schools) has access to an educational psychologist, and in the process of assessing your child's needs you may be asked to give consent for your child to see one. Unfortunately, most educational psychologists have no special training in dealing with multiples. As a minimum, twins and higher multiples should be assessed on different days and the reports about them written on different days too.

It is not often possible for the educational psychologist to see your twin or twins regularly and you may need to involve other resources, for instance family therapy. You can get guidance on educational issues from Tamba.

You may have heard of 'statementing'. This refers to a statement of special educational needs, and is a term which educational psychologists (and verbal purists) often point out isn't a verb. Briefly, a statement of special educational needs describes the problem in question (along with any non-educational needs), identifies the objectives and outlines the provision to be made to meet them. As a parent, you have the chance to read the statement and comment on it.

A statement of special educational needs is usually drawn up from age two onwards, but it can be done much earlier if need be, for instance if a child has Down's.

The statement carries no stigma or long-term implication.

It doesn't label a child so much as define his needs in an attempt to meet them. Even so, some parents worry about a statement, or about the fact that one of their twins may have been 'statemented' and not the other. If you are concerned about it, just ask yourself, what would be the implications of not getting help for your child's special needs?

· *When a Twin Dies* ·

The death of both twins is self-evidently a tragedy and it is easy to recognise it as one. We normally expect to live longer than our children, so, like all deaths in childhood, it is 'wrong' because it is the wrong way round.

> *Both my twins died within 15 hours of birth. For a long long time I felt something inside had died too. It was me.*

The loss has to be lived through, worked though and ultimately, perhaps many years later, accepted – although, as the columnist Virginia Ironside has put it, you do not really work through bereavement. It works through you.

Tragic though the death of both twins is, it involves none of the conflicting emotions that parents endure when they lose one of their multiples and others survive.

The rest of this section focuses on the loss of one twin (or triplet), not because the death of both (or all) babies is any less important but because the family issues are complex.

First of all, the survivor acts as a constant reminder of the loss – and how can the family celebrate his life while coping with his twin's death? Second, the parents need to look after him, no matter how deep their grief. Third, many well-meaning people fail to understand the extent of the parents' bereavement and often think that a mother who has lost a twin should be content to have one remaining child.

The work done in this field at the Multiple Births Foundation (MBF) as well as in Australia, the USA and elsewhere shows that the loss of one twin, far from being easier on the parents, as many people might expect, is actually harder to bear because parents need to care for the surviving twin and carry on with family life. This postpones the essential process of mourning, as when a pregnancy swiftly follows a still birth or infant death, only more so.

Unfortunately, even those medical professionals who should be of most help to parents who lose one twin have been known to misunderstand, and make hurtful comments which betray an archaic attitude of 'least said, soonest mended'. Not surprisingly, parents of a dead twin tend to talk less about their grief to professionals than do those who lose a singleton.

Yet these parents' needs may be greater. Research suggests that mothers who lose one newborn twin are at higher risk from mental ill-health a year later than those who lose their only child. Another study shows that a parent who loses a twin at birth is more likely to feel hostile, confused and angry than one who loses a singleton.

Part of the grief, according to bereaved parents, is due to the loss of the pride and specialness that goes with twins or higher multiples in the family. A mother, one of whose twins has died, continues to think of herself as a mother of twins, as Elizabeth Bryan has pointed out, and this may need to be acknowledged. Similarly, a mother of triplets, one of whom has died, is still a mother of triplets – she is not somehow relegated to the rank of mother of twins.

Unresolved parental grief is hard on the surviving children, especially the co-twin, who also goes through complex emotional reactions (discussed later in this chapter). A grieving mother may find the demands of childcare overwhelming and be unable to give her best to the surviving twin, but grieve she and her partner must, going through the various stages in the ways which are most appropriate for them. If you are in this situation, the best advice would be to respect the enormity of your loss and try not to rush the grief process.

James Hollis, a Jungian psychotherapist, writes in his book *The Middle Passage* that grief in general is the occasion for acknowledging the value of what has been experienced. Because it has been experienced, it cannot be wholly lost. It is there, says Hollis, retained in the bones and the memory, to serve and guide the life to come.

Experience of the dead twin seems to be an essential part of coming to terms with the loss. When a twin is stillborn or dies as a very young baby, the loss is no less real, but there will have been little opportunity to experience him in life. What then can one keep in the bones and the memory to honour the lost child and the lost twinship?

Death before birth

Even when a baby dies before birth, there are still ways in which parents can mark his existence.

- You could have a photo reproduced from an ultrasound scan, preferably an early one when both babies were alive, but if not, any scan that shows both together.
- Although staff might not think of it, you may want to see, and perhaps hold, the dead twin at delivery. If you and your partner want time alone with the baby, say so. You may wish to hold both babies together.
- Photographs or paintings often become treasured mementoes. Many firms can create a family group from two or more separate photos. Computer imaging helps. When a twin dies long before delivery you may not consider photos to be suitable for showing to others, but sometimes an artist can produce an attractive composite sketch or painting from separate photographs of babies (or even fetuses).

- Naming the dead baby makes it easier for the family to talk about her. Perhaps you could avoid a name which too obviously matches the survivor's (e.g. Daisy and Rose).
- You may be able to arrange a funeral service.
- Even after the body has been disposed of, some priests are prepared to baptise stillborn babies (occasionally even babies who technically miscarried). This can be a great solace to parents. Strictly speaking, this is a baptism 'by intent', and the normal certificate of baptism is issued with those two words added.
- You can hold some kind of memorial service. It does not need to take place straight away – it can be many years later.
- You could mark the existence of the twin in some other tangible way, for instance in the hospital's memorial book, or by planting a tree or inscribing a plaque.
- You and your partner shouldn't avoid discussing your baby together as a couple and with friends and relatives. In due course you will also need to talk to your surviving twin.

Most of these suggestions apply no matter when in pregnancy the twin's death occurred, although there is a particular complication with the death of one baby early in pregnancy. When a twin dies before 24 weeks (or is selectively terminated) while the other continues to term, legally this is considered a miscarriage. However, many parents find it comforting to have both babies registered as twins and this is often possible if you ask.

Death of a young baby or child

This often takes place in hospital, especially in the Special Care Baby Unit, where staff may be experienced in dealing with bereaved parents, though perhaps less adept at handling the death of one twin.

When a twin or higher multiple is dying, parents should try to spend as much time with this baby as possible. There will be plenty of time later with the surviving infant(s). Few staff appreciate this at the time and may suggest that a mother concentrate on the healthier of the two. Yet later parents often wish that they had held and looked after the sicker baby more, instead of letting nurses relieve them of his care.

There are many ways in which a parent can mark and commemorate the existence of the baby:

- Photographs help, preferably of both or all the babies together. Even after one has died, photos can be taken of them together if you want. There are few medical reasons why this should not be done. This sometimes shocks nursing staff, but parents don't usually find it macabre.
- Other useful mementoes are hospital wrist or ankle tags, cot cards, locks of hair and even footprints or fingerprints. You may not appreciate their value now, or even want to look at them, but as time passes little things like these can become treasured possessions.
- Some hospitals have a memorial book in which to inscribe details of the baby.
- As always, naming the baby facilitates talking about him now and in the years to come, not least with the surviving twin when the time comes.
- If you have a same-sex pair, zygosity determination can enable you to know for sure whether they are identical (monozygotic). This can sometimes be arranged if you ask early on.
- Keeping in touch with hospital staff may be your only contact with people who knew your baby in life.
- Writing about your baby and your loss can be a kind of therapy. It could take the form of poetry, prose, diary or letters. You don't have to send the letters.

Help for bereaved families

Many mothers who lose a baby or child are advised to get over it by trying again for another baby as soon as possible. However, pregnancy and birth, being the antitheses of death, inhibit proper mourning. Although the next baby is usually much cherished – and much worried about – rushing into another pregnancy tends to be a poor idea, even when the entire set of twins or triplets was lost.

Parents who lose a child often blame themselves, even though there's very rarely anything they could have done to prevent the tragedy. Blame is useless, but it's nonetheless normal as one tries to make sense of what happened.

Fortunately, help is available to families who lose one or all of their multiple-birth children. Tamba's Bereavement Support Group was set up by and for such families, including those who have suffered a cot death and those who go through complete loss of an assisted pregnancy. The BSG newsletter is a forum for views and many bereaved parents have found that writing for it has crystallised their feelings and helped them come to terms with events. Tamba Twinline takes calls from parents with a variety of queries, including those in the acute distress of bereavement. Parents and professionals can also contact MBF about bereavement.

As in most childcare issues, men tend to be sidelined or at least under-represented. Although help is offered to fathers too, mothers find it easier to avail themselves of it. Sometimes a father's reaction is at odds with his partner's over their loss, but either way it is hard for him to express how he feels. Even in these supposedly caring times, there are few acceptable ways for men to open up. Back at work, colleagues may not think of raising the topic with a bereaved father or asking how things are. And he may not want to burden friends and family. After all, real men don't cry. Or do they?

· *The Surviving Twin* ·

Children feel emotions acutely, and the long-term effects of death on a surviving child, especially the co-twin, can be devastating. This shouldn't be surprising. The link between twins is often the strongest of all human bonds.

Even those who lose a twin in very early childhood can be deeply affected. Strange as it may seem, a few people whose co-twin was stillborn have remarked that they'd always felt incomplete – long before they ever knew they were a twin. Sometimes, a child who is a surviving twin keeps playing with toys that are incomplete, such as a car with a missing wheel, or a teddy bear with only one eye. They are often relieved when they find out that they once had a twin, if only for a few months of life in the womb.

Experts agree that it is a mistake to try to shield a youngster from a death in the family. Although a child's notion of dying may be unsophisticated, he must be told at some point that he both had and lost a twin, preferably before he hears it from someone else. Parents are often surprised at how well children accept this. The surviving child may be extraordinarily proud of the twinship. Some rush to share the news with their best friend.

If a child is old enough at the time of death, the funeral or memorial service can be an important way to say goodbye. Even very young children can get involved by playing their own special role – choosing a song or hymn, or putting a posy of flowers on the coffin. They should be allowed and encouraged to do so if they want, though they shouldn't be forced to.

Whatever the age at which his twin dies, the survivor may feel guilty. Sometimes it is because he feels he didn't look out for his twin, but it may just be non-specific guilt at having survived. As one girl says of her twin brother's still-birth, she was not expected to live either – which is why, her parents told her, they deliberately gave her an ugly name.

Parents need to be careful not to say anything that could lay any blame on the survivor. It can take a great deal of thought to avoid mentioning overcrowding in the womb, lack of nourishment or, say, the suggestion that if Mum hadn't been distracted by Ben, Amy might not have run into the path of an oncoming car.

Any of these may well have happened, possibly colouring the parents' attitude and emotions. The survivor may feel worthless as well as guilty. This is particularly likely to happen when the survivor of a boy-girl pair is, as far as one or other parent is concerned, the 'wrong' sex.

As only half of the twin pair, a survivor may feel that his value is diminished. Sometimes parents idolise the dead twin, and unconsciously vilify the one who is still alive:

> *Somehow I was made to feel second-rate, even before my brother died (at the age of five). He was always the sickly one, but never complained. I was healthy, lively, and too much trouble – at least from our mother's point of view. I realise now that things were tough for her. I was made to feel even worse after he died because she kept going on and on about how perfect he was, 'not like her'.*

Of course, the survivor's misdemeanours may be only too obvious. The surviving child can be hard to handle when he's going through his own emotional maelstrom. In coping with his own grief and confusion he may do things his parents find distressing, such as talking to his dead twin, taking his place at the dining-table or eating only half the food put in front of him.

Occasionally the surviving twin himself seems to court death, especially if the process has been glorified in any way. One six-year-old boy persisted in standing in the road outside the house; perhaps it is significant that this happened around Easter. His twin had not died in an accident, but, as he explained, he wanted to die so Baby Jesus could take him to his brother.

Whatever caused the death, the mother sometimes demands frequent medical check-ups for the surviving child for fear of losing him too. In the case of an illness like leukaemia, it may seem incredible to parents that the remaining child has escaped his twin's fate – they wonder for how long. Sometimes such concerns are rational, but sometimes they are not.

The surviving child may need the expert help of a child psychiatrist, and referral to a traumatic stress clinic that specialises in youngsters can be appropriate. The parents also need help with their emotions. Left unresolved, their own grief will make things much harder on the child. They may also disagree on how to handle issues, and this can make it more difficult for their surviving twin.

Death is rarely all over and done with, and it does not cancel the twinship. Children usually benefit if the memory of their dead twin is kept alive and in later years are often grateful to their parents for this. Parents shouldn't discourage their children from talking about their dead twin. Some youngsters like to visit the grave at special times to place flowers there or just to think, but it takes tact to do this on appropriate anniversaries without spoiling the survivor's birthday celebrations.

At whatever age death occurred, and despite the parents' best efforts, some survivors still feel like only half of a whole. Perhaps this is a unique feature of twinship.

· *Lone Twins as Adults* ·

I believe that if you started life together, then you were meant to be together.

Research shows that bereaved children in general tend to have a higher risk of later psychiatric illness, especially depression. In the 1980s, psychotherapist Joan Woodward carried out a study specifically on surviving twins. She interviewed 219 adults, some of whom had lost a twin in childhood, while others had been bereaved more recently. Woodward herself had lost her identical sister Pamela at the age of three. Over 80 per cent of the twins in her study rated their response to their twin's death as having had a severe or marked effect on their lives. The death of identical or same-sex twins tended to have more severe consequences. Perhaps surprisingly, those who had lost a twin in infancy or at birth sometimes mourned for life.

Some of the themes which emerged from the study echo those affecting surviving child twins. There was often guilt, for instance at not having been there to protect the twin, and there were sometimes feelings of inadequacy. Survivors felt that however much they achieved in life they could never be good enough for two.

Many adult lone twins had trouble relating to other people. Perhaps they were striving, and inevitably failing, to duplicate the closeness and intensity of the twin bond with someone else. Woodward found that some adult twins were intensely lonely, while others shunned closeness and described themselves as loners.

In 1989, with enthusiastic support from MBF, Joan Woodward founded the Lone Twin Network (LTN), which can be contacted via MBF. (In the USA there is a Twinless Twins Support Group, founded by Raymond Brandt.) The Lone Twin Network has grown to several hundred members and offers support and contact to any lone twin over 18 years old. Some get in touch soon after losing their twin, others many decades later – often after years of bottling up their emotions – by which time they have come to believe they must be weird to feel this way.

At whatever time lone twins hear of LTN, there is often profound relief. Many are amazed to find that they are not alone in feeling bereaved, confused or lost themselves. Finally they can acknowledge the depth of their feelings.

The Lone Twin Network holds annual meetings for those who want to attend, and at some of these various other issues have been highlighted, such as the needs of parents of adult lone twins, and those of other siblings.

The impact of losing a twin in childhood resonates throughout life, but one is not always consciously aware of it. Knowing that I can now make contact with other surviving twins who understand and have had a similar emotional reaction is very reassuring. My parents never spoke about my twin, who died suddenly aged five. I can understand that they must have been in a state of shock and denial for some considerable time and then found all the reminders too painful. The consequence is that I have no mementoes of my brother – just one photograph – and now both my parents are dead. I wonder if this is why I volunteered to create a Book of Remembrance for the Lone Twin Network.

What happens to the twinship is a fascinating if painful question. Because twins are so tightly linked, a lone twin may have difficulty in talking about 'I' instead of 'we'. Some survivors discover that their very identity appears to be under threat. For anyone who has recently been bereaved, catching a glimpse of the dead person out of the corner of one's eye is a common recurrent experience. In the case of a lone twin, looking in a mirror is often a long-term repeated reminder of the hurt. Being mistaken for one's identical twin by others can also be acutely painful.

Faith is a solace for some, especially those with a deep conviction that they will eventually be reunited with their twin, but whatever their religious inclinations, most lone twins find it important to create some sort of memorial. It may be in the concrete sense of a plaque or headstone, or it could be by naming one of their own children after their twin.

For those whose twin was stillborn, obtaining the certificate can be a reassuring and tangible reminder of the co-twin's reality. Normally only parents are entitled to a stillbirth certificate, but as a result of MBF's efforts, an exception can be made so that the surviving twin is allowed to have a copy. All these things can help in dealing with the pain of no longer being a twin.

Chapter Sixteen

ADULT TWINS

Most of the time while we were married and each raising our own families, my twin sister Mary and I lived at opposite ends of the country. Our husbands died within two years of each other, and our families have grown up (Mary's son died at the age of 31). It seemed the obvious thing to move in together, and now we share a bedroom again, just like when we were children. Unlike other widows in their seventies, we're never lonely. We're lucky.

Twins often can't visualise life without their twin, nor can singletons imagine what it might be like to have a twin. Psychologists now appreciate that many adult twins relate to each other in ways which ordinary single-born mortals barely understand.

It's generally agreed there's more to twins than just two people who happened to be born at the same time, but what exactly is it? Some people assume there's an eerie psychic connection between twins – and maybe, just maybe, there is. It's a topic explored in several books, including Peter Watson's *Twins*.

· *How Adult Twins See Themselves* ·

Some twins are no closer than any two siblings, while a few identicals continue to have as adults an intense and exclusive relationship, living together, sharing a bedroom, choosing the same clothes and hairdos, working for the same company and finishing each other's sentences in conversations. Some pairs allocate daily tasks in such a way that only one will buy the newspaper, say, or post letters, and these can become chores that the other twin is unable to perform.

Of course, these are the ones that stand out. Most adult twins seem to fall somewhere between these two extremes. The closest links are often between identical twins, though it is not clear why. Is it purely because they are genetically the same, or because their parents brought them up as one unit on account of their striking physical similarity?

Twins with an antipathy to each other

The world at large expects twins to be somehow complementary to each other, yet for a few pairs, twinship is a constricting experience, and each twin can find it difficult to assert his independence even as an adult. This is especially prone to happen when one twin continually looks to his twin for guidance, something which can be unhealthy for both leader and led.

Most adult twins lead completely normal lives and don't have any more problems than anyone else, but some don't get on well. Reasons include:

- constant fighting
- difficulty in developing their own identities; they may even be indistinguishable in family photographs
- extreme similarities, for example two intolerant people rarely get along
- feeling freakish: after all, the rest of the world is composed overwhelmingly of singletons
- unflattering comparisons: one twin can feel permanently inferior, as did the darker-skinned brother of a mixed-race pair; although he resented it, both boys seemed to take this for granted as the natural order, until they reached adulthood

- parental favouritism: the preferred one tends to blossom while his twin may feel he lives in his shadow.

Even when twins do not get on at all well, casual observers and acquaintances may assume they must, on account of their twinship, be best friends. This can be really hurtful – imagine being constantly mistaken for someone you can't stand!

Occasionally, adult twins describe themselves as 'too close for comfort'. Some dislike the existence of another person who is so similar – after all, there's the saying that we're all different. Twins may find it difficult to be together because they are uninhibited with each other, telling each other things they wouldn't dream of saying to outsiders.

Some continue their rivalry into middle age and beyond, competing in terms of houses and their offsprings' academic or sporting achievements. This can also happen with non-twins, though it tends to be more intense with same-sex twins. The efforts are often doomed to fail, as when one of the pair has a less well-paid job and can't afford the same life-style as his twin.

Being a twin is not an issue

A few pairs seem genuinely not to care either way about their twinship. It is no more and no less than the link between any two siblings. It is just there.

'I like him very much, and we are close,' says one woman of her twin brother, 'but no more close than to anyone else. In fact, I'd say I was closer to my older brother than to my twin.'

Being a twin is fun

Two identical twin girls, now both doctors, still seem to find great pleasure in their twinship, although one is the leader and the other follows. Their voices are especially alike and most people get them mixed up on the phone, though not in person. The younger one seems to find it less fun – she was always the follower.

We're still very close

Many twins find their twinship an enduring source of pleasure and support throughout life. The first person to hear of a twin's successes or failures is usually the co-twin, perhaps because they can be counted on to share the intensity of some of the joys and disappointments. One twin now facing redundancy in her forties finds her non-identical sister, although living in another country, particularly concerned and supportive.

· *Surveys of Twins* ·

There are several collections of twin experiences, such as the one by Mary Rosambeau in the 1980s. A psychology graduate, social worker and mother of twins, she sought the views of hundreds of twins in their teens and beyond. Some of her findings are described in her book *How Twins Grow Up*. Many of those who responded were identical twins, so clearly these had something particular to say, whereas non-identicals may have felt less strongly. This bias – or self-selection – amongst respondents means that percentages and figures are difficult to rely on, but it's still fascinating reading. You may also enjoy *Multiple Voices* by Mary Lowe and Pat Preedy, and *Raising Twins* by Eileen M. Pearlman and Jill Alison Ganon (see Further Reading, page 370).

Some of the advantages twins mention are:

- having a soul-mate
- having someone with whom you can be totally honest
- having someone who understands you, no matter what

- being special
- being popular socially
- protecting each other, and presenting a united front, whether at home, at school or at work
- help with practicalities like household chores and homework
- someone to play tennis or board games with
- the benefits of competition (three female athletes who happen to be triplets give this as one of the major reasons for their perseverance and success).

According to twins themselves, there are also disadvantages:

- being valued purely for the twinship rather than as individuals
- being called 'the twins', or 'twinnies'
- insensitive comparisons, especially in such areas as physical appearance or exam results – 'She's the pretty one,' said one young woman. 'She always was. But I'm now the married one!'
- being responsible in some way for the other twin
- being too dependent on each other
- lack of parental time and attention.

Interestingly, the issues adult twins consider important are much the same as the ones focused on in this book from the child-rearing point of view. Some of them can be altered for the better. Although changing society's preconceptions is a tall order, today's parents are in a good position to be aware of the problems their twins face and to help them get the most from being twins.

Until recently, there was little systematic research, but thanks partly to the International Society for Twin Studies this is changing. Researchers have long believed that the closeness between twins excludes others and may inhibit adult twins from enjoying the wide variety of other relationships. Recent studies now question this. Levels of intimacy are high among twins, but that doesn't necessarily lead to dependence. A project from Canada on twins aged 16 to 73 found that identical twins often nominate each other as their closest friend. But, contrary to expectations, those who seem to be more intimate with their twin don't have significantly less intimacy with other close friends. Intimacy is a part of all important relationships, and feeling connected with one person may even help someone become connected with others. Perhaps it's time to realise that being a twin can actually have a beneficial impact on other close relationships.

· *The Opposite Sex* ·

All the same, an outsider can find it hard to intrude on the closeness of twins. Whether or not the twins are of the same sex, prospective partners may feel that they need to obtain permission from the other twin before a relationship can get serious. Twin (and triplet) girls often say that any boyfriend has to get on well with all of them. The thought of such a vetting procedure can put off many interested males.

René Zazzo believed that twins often marry later than singletons and found that many did not marry at all, perhaps out of a sense of loyalty to the twinship. Therapist Audrey Sandbank points out that expectations regarding marriage can be very high. In fact, many of us, whether twins or singletons, have excessively high expectations of our marriages and partnerships, but for twins it may be particularly unrealistic to assume that they will ever develop any bond as deep as that of twinship.

There is anecdotal evidence that the continuing intimate relationship between twins can make a spouse feel insecure. As one woman says:

I actually introduced my twin brother to his future wife, who was a close colleague of mine. Yet for many years into their marriage it was clear that my sister-in-law was very jealous of me. And it is not as if my brother and I were ever inseparable.

This probably says more about the sister-in-law's assumptions about twins' relationships than it does about these twins.

When only one twin marries or develops a lasting relationship, trouble can result, with the other feeling left on the shelf. It can cause estrangement between the twins. Often the unhappiness is temporary, and in due course the single twin finds his feet and makes his own way. Occasionally the remaining twin hastily finds a partner too, but a distress purchase can be unsuitable.

On the other hand, the twin left behind is sometimes relieved rather than upset at remaining single. After all, the marriage and moving away of one of the pair also eliminates some of the disadvantages of twinship, which can be a liberating experience.

Occasionally there are other unusual facets of twins' relationships with others:

- Young adult twins may play tricks on girlfriends or boyfriends. This 19-year-old did:

  When I was seeing someone I actually didn't like very much, I sent my identical brother once to meet her in my place. She didn't crack it, although she might have done in time. He didn't like her either, as it happens, but he got a kick out of playing this massive trick on her!

- Twins sometimes marry other twins. Exactly why this should happen is not clear, but we do tend to choose as partners people like ourselves.
- Twins, usually same-sex pairs, may be attracted to the

same person. In fact, this seems to happen far less often than one would suppose and possibly slightly less often than it occurs with any singleton siblings. Many twins say they would never find the same person attractive because they have different tastes, but it also could be a form of unspoken taboo akin to incest.

- A few people have sexual relationships with both twins simultaneously. At university one undergraduate alternately bedded two identical sisters for several months, a situation one of them knew about and accepted, while the other one (who happened to be the dominant one of the twinship) was apparently unaware of events. And at least one woman is known to co-habit with identical brothers, all three of them sharing a bedroom and a relationship. When she appeared on television with this story, it was clear that she treated the men as one unit. How serious are such relationships? It is impossible for outsiders to know.

· Did the Parents of Adult Twins · Get It Right?

This question is very relevant to today's parents of multiples. Again, there is no one answer, and there's very little formal research. One can probably generalise from the wealth of anecdotes and observations available that those twins who were helped from an early age to be individuals do best as independent functional adults.

I felt that my mother, who was a single parent for much of our childhood, coped very well and was very wise too. She raised us all as individuals, so that we each grew up to have a sense of our own worth. And I am very grateful for it, because with twins and four other kids it couldn't have been easy.

Psychotherapists say that adulthood experiences sometimes suggest things might have worked out better had parents done things differently:

> *Mum and Dad could probably have done better. I thought our upbringing was normal at the time, but looking back I think our parents were so tickled by having identical twins that they failed to see we needed to develop away from each other as well as from them. We were treated more like Siamese twins. And I think we were treated as babies for far longer than if we'd been single-born because we were so cute. Well, they thought we were.*

All is not necessarily lost, however. Adult twins who are unable to function well independently may benefit from appropriate therapy.

What are today's children likely to think?

Thirty or 40 years ago there was little awareness of the needs of twins and higher multiples, so perhaps it shouldn't be surprising that a few have had enduring problems in adulthood. But things have changed. There are more multiples born, for a start. Medical care has advanced, parenting has become less rigid, and information has never been as accessible as it is today. Taking into account the research now being done into the issues concerning multiples, it may well be that today's youngsters will fare better – psychologically as well as medically – than they would have a couple of decades ago. However, it would be wrong to be complacent about the challenges families face. Audrey Sandbank points out that the kind of twin problems she sees in family therapy are much the same as the ones she dealt with 20 to 30 years ago.

Advice from adult twins

Happily, few of the adult twins I have spoken to are critical of their own parents, but several wanted to pass on advice to mums and dads of young twins. Since the points they make also appear under different headings elsewhere in this book, I apologise for the repetition, but these are important recurring themes.

- Don't dress them alike, or at least only as small babies.
- Give them separate bedrooms as soon as you can – and as soon as they want them.
- Be fair where possible.
- Avoid insensitive (and often pointless) comparisons.
- Help them function separately at school as well as at home.
- Give them the freedom to be themselves.

This last comment is echoed by therapist Audrey Sandbank, who believes that twins should be given choices as they grow up, so that they can make up their own minds about being close or apart.

· *Twin Phenomena* ·

Baby twins put up for adoption are no longer placed with separate families if it can possibly be helped, but at one time they were, often without telling them or their new parents that they were twins. This meant that a number of twins were raised apart, sometimes in very different households and without knowing until much later that they had a twin somewhere. In some cases the twins discovered their twin-ship in adulthood (some suspected it earlier) and made efforts to be reunited with their co-twin.

There have been some uncanny results. The so-called 'Jim twins' from Ohio, USA, are among the best-known examples of amazing coincidental similarities between twins reared apart. Adopted separately in 1939, both were given the forename James by their adoptive families. This is unremarkable, but there were some surprising parallels between them. When they met up around the age of 40, the two Jims found that they both had sons with the same names; they had each married a woman called Linda and later divorced, each to marry a Betty; they had several habits in common, including common ones like nail-biting and more unusual ones like leaving love-notes around the house; they drank the same type of beer, smoked the same brand of cigarettes, had the same hobbies and sporting interests, and suffered from much the same ailments.

For many years psychologists from the University of Minnesota have been studying twins, including those brought up separately. In 1983 Professor Thomas Bouchard Jr established the Minnesota Center for Twin and Adoption Research. It has several aims and functions: some are educational, while others include helping those still trying to find their co-twin. The Center is based in Minneapolis, which is in itself interesting. Minneapolis and the adjoining town of St Paul have long been known as the Twin Cities for geographical reasons. Minneapolis is bigger, though St Paul is the dominant twin in that it is the state capital of Minnesota.

Twins reared apart can give useful insights into the relative importance of nature and nurture, and also raise questions about the possibility of extra-sensory perception (ESP) or psychic communication. The Minnesota Study of Twins Reared Apart is just one of the Center's projects. In this programme, adult twins are invited to the university for a week of in-depth assessment to elucidate the environmental and genetic factors responsible for various medical and psychological characteristics.

Some of the similarities found when twins meet up have

been striking, as in the case of the Jim twins, but a few could be simply coincidental. What, for instance, is the probability of two unrelated people wearing similar clothes on a cold day? Clearly there is a likelihood that they might just have chosen the same coat by chance, especially if it is of a type widely available. If you shop at Marks & Spencer, for instance, you won't have to go far to find someone else – probably of similar age to yourself – wearing the same garment.

It could be that when twins show these similarities people seize on them and call them significant, but other coincidences might be conveniently ignored because they are not interesting enough. This topic is outside the scope of this book, but it has been nicely covered in Peter Watson's *Twins*, where you can find out more about the Jim and other reunited twins, as well as other popular aspects of Professor Bouchard's work.

· *Twin Studies* ·

Twins offer a powerful research method for understanding the relative importance of genes and the environment in health and disease, as well as in complex human traits. It complements the work done in gene sequencing, for instance the Human Genome Project. Twin research demands meticulous data-handling and a high level of participation by twins and their families, who have to be prepared to give their time and effort.

There are now many twin registers around the world and they focus on different areas of study. Some registers are vast, others much smaller, allowing researchers to go into the kind of detail that would be impossible on a larger scale. The huge St Thomas' UK Adult Twin Register was started in London in 1993. It has grown to include around 10,000 people aged 18 to 80 from all over the UK. Areas of research include osteoporosis, osteoarthritis, blood pressure, heart disease, eczema, acne, hay fever as well as cataracts and other forms of eye disease. These are fascinating and potentially useful projects, to which identical and non-identical twins can contribute if they are interested (contact details are on page 375).

Identical twins (or to be more exact, monozygotic – MZ – twins) are genetically indistinguishable, so any differences between them are due to the environment. It sounds straightforward enough, but the classic twin study method has complicating factors which researchers need to take into account. For instance:

- Even if two people have the same genes, the genes aren't necessarily expressed in exactly the same way. A gene can, in effect, lie dormant. We know this happens with the X chromosome, for instance.
- Being brought up together or living together for a long time makes people similar in many ways – both physically and psychologically – so that some similarities between identical twins reared together may be due to their shared environment. Ignore this factor and you could over-estimate the importance of genetics.
- The pre-birth environment can be very different even for identical twins.

So far, there have been many interesting answers to old questions, and, as with all the best research, a crop of fascinating new questions to excite generations to come.

Appendix

· *Chorionicity* ·

One very important use of ultrasound is to establish what is known as chorionicity: whether twins in the womb have two chorionic membranes or just one. Most twins have two and are called dichorionic, while a minority will be monochorionic (see also pages 22–24).

There is a difference between zygosity (identicalness) and chorionicity, even though not all midwives or doctors realise it! All non-identicals (dizygotic or DZ) and about one-third of identicals (monozygotic or MZ) are dichorionic, leaving the remainder monochorionic.

Whether identical twins turn out to be monochorionic or dichorionic depends on when the fertilised ovum splits into two:

- If it happens within three days of fertilisation, the twins are dichorionic.
- If the ovum splits after three days, the twins are monochorionic.

How can one tell?

When the twins are dichorionic, a small wedge-shaped area (called the lambda sign) shows up between the two sacs on scans between 10 and 14 weeks of pregnancy. It's sometimes seen a bit later on too, but not always.

Why does it matter?

Many of the twin pregnancies which do less well are monochorionic, with twin-to-twin transfusion syndrome (see below) being the main problem. If there is only one chorion, it's therefore wise to monitor the pregnancy more closely, with scans every two weeks from 16 to at least 24 weeks. Sometimes, a mum expecting monochorionic twins is referred to a different maternity unit with greater expertise. Meanwhile if your twin pregnancy is dichorionic, as most are, you can be reassured that you and your babies fall into a low-risk group. Most hospitals now assess chorionicity in twin and higher-order pregnancies.

Are your twins monochorionic?

Unless your hospital assesses chorionicity with an early scan, you may not be sure, but your twin pregnancy is definitely dichorionic – so relatively low-risk – if either:

- the placentas are separate, or
- you have a boy-girl pair.

· Twin-to-Twin Transfusion Syndrome · (TTTS) or Feto-Fetal Transfusion Syndrome

This is a rare but dangerous complication of some identical (monozygotic or MZ) twin pregnancies. It affects those which have only one chorion (see above).

About 80 per cent of all monochorionic placentas have interconnecting blood vessels. Trouble crops up if blood is shunted from one baby to the other; it's effectively a blood transfusion (hence the name of the condition). TTTS often works out badly for both babies.

What can happen?

The so-called donor ends up giving blood to his twin. As the pregnancy continues, he becomes much smaller, anaemic, possibly shrivelled and may have disabilities.

Meanwhile, the recipient, who gets more of the blood, is larger and redder. He may have heart failure and will usually produce more amniotic fluid, resulting in polyhydramnios. In fact a woman's discomfort from polyhydramnios is often the first sign that something is amiss. (For more on poly-hydramnios, see Chapter 2.)

That is what happens in full-blown TTTS. Happily, many babies are affected only to a mild extent and may just show some discrepancy in size or colouring. It is said that the biblical twins Jacob and Esau may have had TTTS, which would explain why Jacob was so pale and Esau so red.

Sometimes there are very few symptoms until after the birth, when labour pumps more blood into the recipient twin. This can even lead to brain damage. For this reason, a caesarean is best if there's any degree of TTTS.

It is likely that around 15 per cent of monochorionic pregnancies overall – or about one in every 30 twin preg-nancies – are affected by TTTS to some degree because of their blood-vessel interconnections.

Making the diagnosis

If your twins are monochorionic, the pregnancy can be monitored regularly by USS for signs of TTTS. Your specialist will be looking out for differences in the size of the twins' abdomens, differences in estimated birth weights, large discrepancies in the amount of amniotic fluid (the donor twin often has very little amniotic fluid while the recipient has a lot) and a discrepancy in the volume of their bladders (the recipient twin may have a much larger bladder because he is carrying more fluid).

What if you don't know the chorionicity, perhaps because your hospital doesn't check for this? If there are two placentas, or the babies are of different sexes, you can stop worrying right away – your babies are dichorionic and won't get TTTS.

If you still don't know the chorionicity, don't panic, but look out for early symptoms like discomfort or a rapidly expanding belly. Get your doctor or midwife to take any symptoms of this sort seriously, to prevent the consequences of severe untreated TTTS. Make a fuss if you have to. TTTS is still rare and there may be one or two professionals who know little about this condition. You would not easily forgive them – or yourself – if you lost your twins because you didn't get the right attention in time.

Treatment

Unfortunately, severe TTTS can be fatal for the babies, but there are several ways of treating it. The main methods are:

- Amniodrainage, which involves drawing off quantities of amniotic fluid by amniocentesis at about weekly intervals.
- Laser treatment of the interconnecting blood vessels, which blocks off the cross-channels. It is done using a fine laser probe between 15 and 28 weeks of pregnancy.

Other treatments include using the heart drug digoxin, and septostomy, which involves making openings between the twins' sacs, so that they effectively have only one amniotic cavity.

Most treatments are carried out under local anaesthetic,

but sometimes laser treatment needs a general anaesthetic. So far, laser therapy may have the edge. Even in severe cases, it seems to give a 70 per cent chance of at least one healthy baby and a 50 per cent chance of two healthy babies. However, the gold standard for evaluating treatments is a randomised controlled trial, and there haven't been any yet in TTTS. To complicate things, published studies of the different treatments have so far included pregnancies with very different degrees of TTTS. If you are unlucky enough to develop the condition, the best option is to discuss it thoroughly with your obstetrician. If you're not already attending a centre specialising in what's known as fetal medicine, you should be referred to one. More information and support is available from the TTTS Foundation (*www.tttsfoundation.org*) or from the UK TTTS Association (*www.twin2twin.org*), which also has a list of UK treatment centres.

· *Selective Termination* ·

Also known as selective birth or selective feticide, this refers to selectively terminating the life of one fetus of a twin (or triplet) pregnancy, while leaving the remaining one(s) intact.

Although it has been done since the late 1970s for a variety of serious disorders, selective termination is not something the average couple knows about. In fact, the first time most people are likely to hear of it is when one of their babies is diagnosed as having a severe or even lethal malformation. This in itself is an extremely distressing discovery to make at a highly emotional time. Taking in new facts and figures is particularly hard at such moments and yet before long the couple will have to make a major decision based on what they understand and how they feel about the situation.

In a twin pregnancy where only one baby is found to have an abnormality, the choice is really three-way:

1 The pregnancy can continue without intervention, in the knowledge that one baby may be born severely disabled. In some cases, the healthy baby may even be put at risk from continuing to share a womb with his twin, not because the condition is in any way catching, but because the abnormal baby may have a mechanical effect. This can happen especially in cases of anencephaly (a very severe skull malformation).
2 The entire pregnancy can be terminated, with the loss of a presumed healthy baby along with the sick one.
3 The pregnancy can be selectively terminated. (For those of you who want technical details, see the section below entitled 'The procedure itself'.)

Occasionally, it's possible for surgeons to correct a baby's abnormalities before birth. Fetal surgery has advanced a lot, though its exact value is still unclear.

The decision

Guided by your specialist, you and your partner have to decide together on the right course of action in the light of the exact diagnosis. A baby who is unlikely to live long after birth may be agonising to bear, but poses different problems from the baby who grows up in constant pain or who becomes a heavy burden to his parents, and to his twin, perhaps for decades. Ask your doctor as many questions as you need to, and jot down the answers so you can remember them later.

Your own religious beliefs and family situation, including any children you have already, also come into the equation. The doctor cannot decide for you, but can provide the information you need and perhaps also act as a sounding-board for your thoughts. Seeing an independent counsellor can help clarify your feelings. Your doctor's own beliefs should not influence your decision. Should your doctor object on principle to selective (or any other) termination, you are entitled to be referred without delay to someone else.

Close family and friends may be very supportive, but they don't always understand the mixed feelings which are natural in this situation. It's hard for some people to grasp that anyone left with one surviving baby (which is all most pregnancies produce, after all) could be hankering for anything more. If you want, your specialist or the MBF can probably put you in touch with another couple who have gone through this experience.

The procedure itself

Selective termination is carried out between 18 and 22 weeks of pregnancy or later. The main time constraint against acting earlier is that the abnormality probably won't have been picked up before 18 weeks.

First, an ultrasound has to establish that the fetuses each have their own placental circulation. If they are monochorionic (see page 23) they will share a blood flow and selective termination carries a high risk of both babies dying as a result. However, some centres may be able to take this on.

In selective termination, a scan is used to locate the abnormal fetus and his placenta. Under ultrasound control, a fine needle is carefully passed through the woman's abdomen and into the affected baby. An injection of local anaesthetic is given; this is 100 per cent successful and works immediately.

The remaining baby is then checked just to make sure he's still well. If you are rhesus negative, you will need an injection of anti-D at this stage to prevent complications of rhesus incompatibility, exactly as if you had just delivered a baby.

Immediately afterwards, you may lose the sensation of kicking from that part of your belly. Over the next few weeks, the dead fetus shrinks dramatically, though there will usually be some evidence of it at delivery.

What about the other baby? There is believed to be a miscarriage rate of 5 to 10 per cent for the survivor. The later the procedure is done, the greater the risk seems to be, so you'll have frequent scans to monitor the remainder of your pregnancy.

More than 20 years' experience of selective termination in centres all over the world suggests that the presence of the dead fetus alongside the survivor causes few physical problems. In fact, the situation seems to resemble the many cases where nature causes one baby of a multiple pregnancy to perish before birth. Premature labour appears to be a risk, but this is a hazard of twin pregnancy anyway, and it's not clear that the risk is significantly greater after selective termination.

You may be wondering about pain. The question of whether – or rather when – a fetus can feel pain is a difficult one. Pain sensation requires connections between certain parts of the brain, like the thalamus and the cortex, and these develop fairly late. It's likely that fetuses can begin to feel pain in the second part of the pregnancy, probably from 23 weeks onwards. This is why, in 1991, the Royal College of Obstetricians and Gynaecologists recommended that from 24 weeks of pregnancy doctors carrying out procedures or terminations should consider the need for pain relief and sedation. In the case of selective terminations, almost all are done before then.

Emotions

It is entirely normal to feel sad and to grieve for your lost baby – even for your lost role as a parent of twins. Your reaction may not be obvious right away. For example, it may not be until your healthy surviving baby is born that you fully appreciate your bereavement. By then other people, including some midwives and doctors, may consider that you should somehow have 'got over it' and be concentrating on looking after your live baby. They do not mean to be thoughtless, but that's how it can come across.

You may indeed be able to put your loss behind you, but this isn't possible for everyone. Unresolved grief can make it an uphill struggle to go on with normal life and especially with caring for a baby who should, had all been well, have had a healthy companion born alongside him.

It may help you, as it has others, to acknowledge in tangible ways your lost baby as an individual:

- Perhaps you'll want to see him at the time of delivery. If so, ask in advance. Staff may just assume that you don't.
- You may later want to have a photo of the fetus, or perhaps a painting or a copy of an ultrasound picture. If you don't want to see your dead baby at delivery, you may still want someone to take a photo, just in case.
- Giving your dead baby a name will help identify him and could help you and your partner talk about him more easily. Remember that, as with two live-born twins, it may be kinder on your surviving baby not to have a matching name.
- A funeral or memorial service can be arranged if you wish.
- Counselling may help you and your partner come to terms with what happened. Contact your GP, ARC (Antenatal Results and Choices; see Resources, page 372) or MBF if you would like support, or get in touch with Tamba Bereavement Support Group.

Before long, you will need to tell your surviving child about his co-twin. The long-term emotional effects of selective termination on a survivor aren't yet known, but it's probably best to be open with the rest of the family. Things have a habit of coming out and you wouldn't want him to find out from someone else. Even without being told of their twinship, surviving lone twins can somehow be acutely aware that they had a companion before birth (there's more on this subject in Chapter 15).

Of course, you don't have to give a child details of how his twin died – just the information that he was very sick and didn't live long enough to be born. This requires a great deal of sensitivity. The survivor may need reassurance that he was not to blame in any way for what happened.

· *Fetal Reduction in Higher-order* · *Multiple Pregnancies*

This is also called multifetal pregnancy reduction. In this procedure, a triplet, quadruplet, or even higher-order pregnancy is reduced to a twin (or even singleton) pregnancy to reduce the risk of disability and thus increase the chances of producing a healthy baby. Many parents and even some family doctors won't have heard of it, but specialists have been doing this procedure since the 1980s in many countries around the world. Research shows that reducing quads (and triplets) to twins now gives an outcome as good as that for a pregnancy which was twins all along. The technique is described below under 'The procedure itself' for those who want to know how it's done.

Pregnancy reduction is a highly complex and emotive issue, and there are many ethical considerations. You won't want to contemplate it at all if you have conscientious objections to termination. Even among doctors who do terminations there are many different shades of opinion.

Some obstetricians believe there can never be any justification for reducing a pregnancy which is progressing well, no matter how many embryos there are. On the other hand, many specialists consider that reducing triplet pregnancies to twins is perfectly rational and justifiable since triplets do less well. A few would even offer to reduce a twin pregnancy since single babies fare better. After all, one at a time is the normal way humans come into the world.

Most obstetricians fall somewhere in the middle, especially since the outlook for twins and triplets is improving. They would be prepared to reduce a quad, quin or sextuplet pregnancy on the basis that carrying fewer fetuses can increase the 'take-home' baby rate. The specialist's own experience of caring for multiple pregnancies can obviously be relevant too.

The decision

Only you and your partner can decide what's right for your circumstances and the limitations of your resources – social, emotional and financial – and you have to decide without the benefit of hindsight. It is a gamble and time constraints add to the pressure. If you do nothing, you could end up with a number of beautiful healthy babies, or you could lose some or all. Quads and more do face a higher risk of death or disability, mainly because the babies are more likely to be both small and premature. But knowing this is not the same as actually making a choice. Nothing about the decision is easy and prospective parents need to talk it over between themselves and with someone else. Some couples only discuss it with the doctor who would carry out the procedure, and this isn't ideal as they can feel pressurised (a few couples decide to get a second medical opinion at this stage). There's certainly a place for a counsellor in this process, and most units can arrange this. Having said that, a few parents are so troubled with the enormity of the whole issue that they actually prefer their specialist to take the lead in arriving at a decision.

The procedure itself

If you go ahead, fetal reduction is done between 11 and 13 weeks. This applies even if you had treatment for infertility, and therefore knew from very early on how many babies there were. It's usually worth waiting till 12 weeks not only to give yourselves time to decide, but because there is some risk of natural pregnancy loss before then. A few specialists carry out pregnancy reduction at seven weeks, though that leaves a couple less time to make up their minds.

The choice as to which fetuses to terminate is generally made on technical grounds, depending on which are most accessible. Otherwise the principles are much the same as for selective termination, described earlier in this Appendix.

Guided by ultrasound, a needle is passed through the woman's abdomen and into the fetus's chest and local anaesthetic is then injected. This works immediately. If many fetuses are to be terminated, the procedure is sometimes done in two stages a week or so apart. Fetal reduction can also be done through the woman's cervix, but this is less common.

Technically, the success rate approaches 100 per cent and complications are unusual. You'll have frequent scans afterwards to keep an eye on progress for the rest of the pregnancy. There are few physical side-effects apart from a risk of miscarriage, but research suggests this is no higher than the miscarriage risk in most multiple pregnancies. The outcome of pregnancy reduction is now much better than it once was, so these days there's a far lower risk of miscarriage or very premature birth.

Because the procedure is done early on in a pregnancy, there is less to see at delivery than with selective termination.

Emotions

An element of sadness or even guilt, no matter how unfounded, may tinge the rest of your pregnancy. You and your partner may feel uneasy at having terminated one or more fetuses, especially as the 'choice' as to which survived has to be made more or less arbitrarily. It may help you to talk things over, perhaps with a counsellor. You can discuss this with Tamba, MBF or your GP.

Many pregnancies of triplets and more result from assisted-reproduction techniques, a fact which saddens and angers some parents and their doctors. It would obviously be better to have avoided these very high-order pregnancies in the first place, for instance by closer monitoring of the effects of fertility treatments. In choosing fetal reduction, however, you may substantially increase your chance of achieving your aim: having at least one healthy baby of your own. Research from the USA suggests that 96 per cent of families who opted for fetal reduction would make the same decision again. Most mothers may feel guilt and grief to begin with, but few have any serious problems after a year, and there's no evidence of any long-term mental distress.

What do you eventually tell your surviving child or children? You might want to tell a child that he was originally one of quads, say, but the knowledge that you terminated his companions would be extremely difficult to bear. It could be agonising to grow up thinking that, but for chance, you could have died instead. To date there's no published research on how surviving children cope. Perhaps it is better to keep a pregnancy reduction secret. To be on the safe side, that means nobody other than the mother and father (and their doctor) should know about it. This obviously makes it harder for a parent, but it could be the best option.

· Cot Death (Sudden Infant Death · Syndrome)

Cot death (SIDS) is the sudden unexpected death of a baby for no obvious reason. It is rarer than it was, but it is slightly more common in twins and multiple births, at least in those that are premature or low in birth-weight. Of course, the vast majority of small babies survive the first year without mishap so you needn't worry too much, but it is worth knowing about cot death and what you can do to reduce the risk.

Cot death affects babies under a year old and mostly under six months. Slightly more boys than girls have cot deaths. Although nobody really knows the cause, overheating and overwhelming infection – to which new babies lack immunity – are probably important. Research has highlighted measures to prevent some cot death and these seem to be working. In the UK, SIDS has become 70 per cent less common following a 1991 government campaign giving advice to parents on the sleeping position of young babies and other matters. All the same, about seven babies a week die from cot death in the UK.

What you can do to reduce the risk

- Always place your babies on their backs to sleep unless your doctor has given you a specific reason not to. The side will do too, though a baby may roll on to his front unless you extend the underneath arm. Don't use wedges or rolled-up towels. Once your babies can move about and choose their own sleeping positions, they are generally out of the cot death danger period.
- Make sure the babies' heads cannot get completely covered by bedclothes. This means putting them in the 'feet to foot' position, so that each baby's feet touch

the foot of the cot, with the blankets firmly tucked in at the bottom and made up no higher than his shoulders. If you put your twins to sleep together, make sure the covers aren't loose as this might allow the head of one or other twin to get covered.

- Don't smoke, either during or after pregnancy, and make sure your partner doesn't smoke either. Keep your babies out of smoky atmospheres and ask visitors not to smoke in the house.

- Don't let your babies become overheated. The ideal room temperature is around 65°F (18°C). Buy a room thermometer if necessary. Unless the weather is exceptionally cold, central heating can usually be turned off at night. If you swaddle your babies, use lightweight materials and leave their heads uncovered. Swaddling is instead of blankets – with blankets as well a baby can get dangerously hot. If you use sleep-sacks, they should be the kind suitable for regular indoor night use, and without a hood. Each baby would need his own bag, and it must be the right size to prevent him from sliding down it, and again getting his head covered.

- Never overdress your babies, especially if they're ill or running a fever. Avoid hot-water bottles and electric blankets altogether. Sheepskins are probably all right as long as your babies sleep on their backs, but avoid them when they start rolling over.

- Don't let very young babies get too cold, either. They need to be wrapped up outside in cold weather.

- The safest place for a baby to sleep for the first six months is in a cot in your bedroom. Finding room for two (or more) cots can be hard, so this might be a reason for your babies to share a cot. You should not have your babies in bed with you, especially if you or your partner are smokers (no matter where you smoke), have been drinking alcohol, take any drugs that make you drowsy, or feel very tired (see also Chapter 6). With twins you also have to make sure one or other baby can't fall out.

- Routine immunisation significantly lowers the risk of cot death.
- In some countries such as New Zealand, cot-death campaigns have advocated breast-feeding as a preventive measure. It may help protect against cot death, but there is no proof of this.
- If you suspect one of your babies is unwell, get medical advice.

Parents sometimes ask about apnoea alarms, which are designed to go off if a baby stops breathing momentarily. Current medical opinion is that these alarms are not in themselves enough to save lives that might have been lost to cot death. They can give false alarms or, on occasion, fail to sound and give a false sense of reassurance. Although apnoea alarms can be helpful, they should not be used without medical supervision.

You should phone 999 or go straight to hospital (accident and emergency department) if a baby:

- stops breathing
- turns blue
- is very drowsy or unrousable.

After a cot death

If there has been a cot death in your family, you will no doubt worry about whether it could happen to the surviving twin. It is very rare for the second twin to die just after the first, but all the same he will almost certainly be taken into hospital immediately for a few days' observation to make sure he remains healthy.

There is also a slightly higher risk of cot death in any baby you have later. In the UK, a programme called CONI (Care of the Next Infant) provides support for the subsequent baby and can help identify those at extra-high risk.

Cot death is rare but is without doubt a devastating experience. As a parent, you will want to know why it happened, but it is not always possible to give an answer. Although it is understandable that you may want to go through and analyse your baby's last few days and hours, try not to blame yourself.

In the case of twins or more, there are also other complex issues surrounding infant death (see Chapter 15). You can get help from Tamba Bereavement Support Group and the Foundation for the Study of Infant Deaths (see page 373).

· *Attention Deficit Disorder* ·

Attention deficit disorder (ADD) is also known as hyper-activity or, more accurately, attention deficit hyperactivity disorder (ADHD). The term ADHD is the one used in the USA, but it's gaining ground in the UK because it's a good description of the main symptoms.

ADHD probably exists all over the world, but its diagnosis is much more readily accepted in the USA and Australia. It may be overdiagnosed in some countries but it is almost certainly underdiagnosed here. In the UK, ADHD tends to be put in the same category as dyslexia, chronic fatigue syndrome and food allergies: all conditions which are hard to prove and sometimes blamed on overactive middle-class imaginations. Furthermore, resources for children and young adults with ADHD are poor, so those who have this very real condition can miss out on treatment.

Who has it?

ADHD is thought to affect about 5 per cent of all children, depending on whether or not one counts mild cases. Boys usually outnumber girls by a factor of three to one. Genetics are important – a sibling of someone with ADHD has a 30 to 40 per cent chance of being affected too, while if one identical twin has it, the other will also have it in 90 per cent of cases.

Twins have a particularly high incidence anyway. Professor David Hay from Australia found ADHD to be nearly twice as common in twins as in singletons. The twin–singleton difference exists in both sexes, but ADHD is more common in boys, and up to 16 per cent of twin boys have it. Twins with reading problems tended to have more ADHD symptoms in this study. Why ADHD is more common in twins is not known, and research continues.

ADHD can run in families from one generation to the next. Grandma may point out that a small child is 'just like his dad was as a youngster'.

Symptoms

There are three main types of ADHD:

- lack of attention
- hyperactivity/impulsivity
- combined type, with a mix of inattention and hyperactivity.

In a child, the typical symptoms are:

- lack of attention and concentration
- overactivity, with constant fidgeting
- disorganisation
- lack of social skills
- clumsiness
- disruptive behaviour.

In mild cases, ADHD can be difficult to define: all young children show these characteristics to some extent. You would not, for instance, expect a five-year-old to be as organised as an adult, nor to be able to concentrate for as long as a university student. Twins seem to have particularly poor powers of concentration, but this may be just because they interrupt and divert each other.

Usually, symptoms of ADHD come to light around the age of two, or else early on in primary school. Occasionally babies who are very active in the womb later turn out to have ADHD.

ADHD can seriously interfere with learning and behaviour and lead to long-term underachievement. Children with ADHD are not stupid, but they cannot concentrate for long and tend to make silly careless mistakes, so they may do badly at school. As perhaps you might guess, the inattention and combined types of ADHD are most likely to lead to learning problems. Some children with ADHD do well except in certain types of work, like project work, which require a high degree of organisation and tidiness.

They're not deliberately naughty either, but their behaviour can be very bad: some children with ADHD have serious behavioural problems. Because they may have difficulty making friends, they may lack self-esteem.

However, a few children with ADHD have added difficulties with language (for example, with speech, understanding long instructions or answering open-ended questions). In some cases there's a connection between ADHD and other conditions such as dyslexia, co-ordination problems and Asperger's syndrome, which may make learning all the more challenging.

Symptoms don't always improve in the teens, and around 60 per cent of ADHD children continue to have problems as adults.

Making the diagnosis

Sometimes the diagnosis is very obvious, or perhaps someone like your GP, health visitor or teacher has suggested it as a possibility. Consulting a paediatrician, child psychiatrist or educational psychologist will usually tell you whether your children have ADHD.

There are some important criteria for diagnosis. Symptoms must have been present for over six months and have started before the age of seven. The child must show symptoms in more than one setting, not for instance just at home or at playgroup. ADHD symptoms must be out of keeping with the child's developmental stage, and impact on normal life, causing distress or impairment.

Clinching the diagnosis is a matter of talking to parents and teachers and observing children, supplemented by special questionnaires such as the Connor's rating scales. There's no laboratory test for ADHD. Special MRI scans can show subtle abnormalities in some parts of the brain, but these are used only in research and it is not yet feasible to scan on a large scale.

There's a lot of controversy about ADHD, which makes it all the more difficult to meet the needs of affected children and their families. It's important for parents and teachers to realise that it does exist, and causes significant distress and often lasting problems. Contrary to what's sometimes said in the media, it's not at all the same as the 'naughty-but-normal' child, and it is not due to inadequate parenting.

What is the cause?

Nobody knows the exact cause of ADHD, but one thing is certain: it is a neuro-developmental disorder. There's some abnormality of brain function, with new research from the US showing reductions in some areas of the brain and an increase in grey matter. ADHD has a large genetic element, although environment may also be important, at least in some cases. With multiples, constant interruptions from each other may be a factor.

Coping with ADHD

Treating ADHD makes all the difference to children and their families. When the main symptoms are controlled, relationships with family and friends improve, and learning is enhanced. In the longer term, there's evidence that treating ADHD reduces the risk of substance abuse and improves job prospects.

Experts generally agree that the best treatment is a combination of behavioural therapy and drug treatment. Unfortunately, child psychiatrists and psychologists are thin on the ground, so it's not always easy to get behavioural treatment (for both child and family). With long waiting-lists, it's best for doctors to refer children as early as possible. The family and school can do a lot, but it's a challenge to love a child just as he is, especially if he's different from his siblings. Youngsters with ADHD can be very demanding and may have few friends, which means their family may be the only source of good feelings. It is important to be loving yet firm in handling and to set clear limits and regular routines. This may not be enough to solve the problem, but it helps. At school, supportive knowledgeable teachers make all the difference.

Drugs for ADHD sometimes have a bad press but they can work well for many children. Most of the medicines are, paradoxically, stimulant drugs like methylphenidate (Ritalin) and dexamphetamine. When they work, their effect can be astonishing, but they do need to be given regularly under the guidance of a specialist. New treatments on the horizon include the non-stimulant drug atomoxetine, already in use in the USA.

Diet is a factor in some cases. Here the blame may lie with one or a few foods, such as some artificial colourings, and taking them out of the diet sometimes helps. In a few cases, a more restricted diet may be useful. However, it is important to be careful with this approach. Putting a growing child on a restricted diet can do more harm than good. If you're going to eliminate more than just the odd item, it's best to see a dietitian. Ask your doctor for a referral.

You can get more information from ADDISS, the national Attention Deficit Disorder Information and Support Service (address on page 372).

FURTHER READING

Ainslie, Ricardo C., *The Psychology of Twinship*, University of Nebraska Press (Nebraska) 1995

Australian MBA Inc & Department of Psychology, La Trobe University, *La Trobe Study – Twins in School*, La Trobe University (Melbourne) 1991

Botting, B.J., Macfarlane, A.J., Price, F.V. (eds.), *Three, Four and More: National Study of Triplet and Higher Order Births*, HMSO (London) 1990

Bryan, Elizabeth, *Twins and Higher Multiple Births: A Guide to Their Nature and Nurture*, Edward Arnold (London) 1992

Bryan, Elizabeth, *Twins, Triplets and More: their nature, development, and care*, MBF (London) 1995

Buckler, John, *The Adolescent Years: The ups and downs of growing up*, Castlemead Publications (Ware) 1987

Carlson, Richard, *Don't Sweat the Small Stuff . . . and it's all Small Stuff*, Hodder & Stoughton (London) 1998

Case, Betty Jean, *Living Without Your Twin*, Tibbutt Publishing (Portland, Oregon) 1993

Case, Betty Jean, *We are Twins, But Who Am I?*, Tibbutt Publishing (Portland, Oregon) 1991

Case, Betty Jean, *Exploring Twin Relationships (Is being a twin always fun?)* Tibbutt Publishing (Portland, Oregon) 1996

Crystal, David, *The Cambridge Encyclopaedia of Language* (2nd ed.), Cambridge University Press (Cambridge) 1997

Farmer, Penelope (ed.), *Two, or The Book of Twins and Doubles: an autobiographical anthology*, Little, Brown (London) 1996

Green, Christopher, and Chee, Kit, *Understanding ADHD: a parent's guide to Attention Deficit Hyperactivity Disorder in Children*, Vermilion (London) 1997

Haslam, David, *Sleepless Children: a handbook for parents*, Piatkus (London) 1992

Kohn, Ingrid, and Moffitt, Perrin-Lynn, *Pregnancy Loss: a Silent Sorrow*, Hodder & Stoughton (London) 1995

Leiter, Gila, *Everything You Need to Know to Have a Healthy Twin Pregnancy*, Dell (New York) 2000

Lowe, Mary, and Preedy, Pat, *Multiple Voices*, The Wine Press (Tamworth, Staffs) 1998

Luke, Barbara, and Eberlein, Tamara, *When You're Expecting Twins, Triplets, or Quads*, HarperCollins (New York) 1999

McFadyen, Anne, *Special Care Babies and their Developing Relationships*, Routledge (London) 1995

Noble, Elizabeth, *Having Twins and More* (3rd ed.), Houghton Mifflin (New York) 2003

Pearlman, Eileen M., and Ganon, Jill Alison, *Raising Twins*, HarperCollins (New York) 2000

Piontelli, Alessandra, *Twins – from fetus to child*, Routledge (London) 2002

Rosambeau, Mary, *How Twins Grow Up*, Bodley Head (London) 1987

Sandbank, Audrey, *Twins and the Family*, Tamba and Arrow Books (London) 1988

Sandbank, Audrey (ed.), *Twin and Triplet Psychology: a professional guide to working with multiples*, Routledge (London) 1999

Segal, Nancy, *Entwined Lives: twins and what they tell us about human behavior*, Dutton (New York) 1999

Spector, Tim, *Your Genes Unzipped*, Robson Books (London), 2003

Stewart, Elizabeth, *Exploring Twins – towards a social analysis of twinship*, Macmillan (London) 2000

Triplets, Quads and Quints Association, *Finding our Way –*

Life with Triplets, Quadruplets and Quintuplets, Multiple Births Canada (Ontario) 2000

Ward, Sally, *Babytalk*, Random House (London) 2000

Watson, Peter, *Twins*, Hutchinson (London) 1981

Woodward, Joan, *The Lone Twin: understanding twin bereavement and loss*, Free Association Press (London), 1998

Wright, Lawrence, *Twins – Genes, Environment, and the Mystery of Identity*, Weidenfeld & Nicolson (London) 1997

RESOURCES

Useful Addresses

Tamba (Twins & Multiple
Births Association)
2 The Willows
Gardner Road
Guildford
Surrey GU1 4PG
Tel. 0870 770 3305
www.tamba.org.uk

Tamba Twinline
Tel. 0800 138 0509 (evenings
and weekends)

MBF (Multiple Births
Foundation)
Queen Charlotte's & Chelsea
Hospital
Hammersmith House Level 4
Du Cane Road
London W12 0HS
Tel. 020 8383 3519
www.multiplebirths.org.uk

Action on Pre-Eclampsia
(APEC)
84–88 Pinner Road
Harrow
Middx HA1 4HZ

Tel. 020 8863 3271
Helpline 020 8427 4217
www.apec.org.uk

ADDISS (the national
Attention Deficit Disorder
Information and Support
Service)
10 Station Road
London NW7 2JU
Tel. 020 8906 9068
www.addiss.co.uk

ARC (Antenatal Results and
Choices) (support around
difficult decisions when an
unborn baby has an
abnormality)
73 Charlotte Street
London W1T 4PN
Tel. 020 7631 0280
Helpline 020 7631 0285
www.arc-uk.org

Association for Post-Natal
Illness
145 Dawes Road
London SW6 7EB

Helpline 020 7386 0868
www.apni.org

BLISS (the premature baby
charity)
68 South Lambeth Road
London SW8 1RL
Tel. 0870 770 0337
Helpline 0500 618140
www.bliss.org.uk

CAPT (Child Accident
Prevention Trust)
18–20 Farringdon Lane
London EC1R 3HA
Tel. 020 7608 3828
www.capt.org.uk

Child Death Helpline
Great Ormond Street Hospital
Great Ormond Street
London WC1N 3JH
Tel. 0800 282986
www.childdeathhelpline.org.uk

Compassionate Friends (for
parents whose children have
died)
53 North Street
Bristol BS3 1EN
Tel. 0117 9539639
www.tcf.org.uk
Contact-a-Family (information
and support for parents of
special-needs children,
including those with rare

disorders)
209–211 City Road
London EC1V 1JN
Tel. 020 7608 8700
Helpline 0808 8083555
www.cafamily.org.uk

CRY-SIS (help for parents of
crying babies)
BM CRY-SIS
London WC1N 3XX
Helpline 020 7404 5011
www.cry-sis.com

Disability Rights Commission
Freepost MID 02164
Stratford-upon-Avon
Warks CV37 9BR
Tel. 0845 7622633
www.drc-gb.org

Doula UK
PO Box 26678
London N14 4WB
www.doula.org.uk

Foundation for the Study of
Infant Deaths
Artillery House
11–19 Artillery Row
London SW1P 1 RT 7DP
Tel. 0870 787 0885 (office)
Helpline 0870 787 0554
www.sids.org.uk
Harris Birthright Research
Centre (research into fetal
medicine and antenatal testing)
9th Floor

Ruskin Wing
King's College School of
Medicine
Denmark Hill
London SE5 8RX
Tel. 020 7924 0894
www.harris-birthright.org

Home Dads (support and
information for stay-at-home
fathers)
www.homedad.org.uk

Home Start UK (national
network of volunteer parents
offering help to families of
young children)
2 Salisbury Road
Leicester LE1 7QR
Helpline 08000 68 63 68
Tel. 0116 2339955
www.home-start.org.uk

International Association of
Infant Massage (IAIM)
PO Box 247
Rainham
Essex RM13 7WT
Tel. 07816 289 788
www.iaim.org.uk

International Society for Twin
Studies (ISTS)
www.ists.qimr.edu.au
La Leche League (advice and
information to women wanting
to breast-feed)
PO Box 29

West Bridgford
Nottingham NG2 7NP
Helpline 020 7242 1278
www.laleche.org.uk

MAMA (Meet-A-Mum
Association; network to
alleviate the isolation of
mothers)
376 Bideford Green
Linslade
Leighton Buzzard
Beds LU7 2TY
www.mama.org.uk

Maternity Alliance (campaigns
for better maternity benefits,
services and rights, and gives
information to pregnant
women at work)
Third Floor West
Northburgh Street
London EC1V 0AY
Tel. 020 7490 7639 (office)
www.maternityalliance.org.uk

Miscarriage Association
c/o Clayton Hospital
Northgate
Wakefield
W. Yorks WF1 3JS
Tel. 01924 200799
www.miscarriageassociation.
org.uk

National Childbirth Trust
(NCT)
Alexandra House

Oldham Terrace
London W3 6NH
Tel. 0870 4448707
www.nctpregnancyandbaby
care.com

National Council for One-
Parent Families
255 Kentish Town Road
London NW5 2LX
Tel. 020 7428 5400
www.oneparentfamilies.org.uk

NHS Direct (24-hour nurse-led
advice on health matters)
Tel. 0845 46 47
www.nhsdirect.nhs.uk

NHS Stop Smoking Helpline
Tel. 0800 169 0 169
www.givingupsmoking.co.uk

Parentline Plus (support for
anyone parenting children)
Helpline 0808 800 2222
www.parentlineplus.org.uk

Royal Society for the
Prevention of Accidents
(RoSPA)
Edgbaston Park
353 Bristol Road
Birmingham B5 7ST
Tel. 0121 248 2000
www.rospa.org.uk

Stillbirth and Neonatal Death
Society (SANDS)
28 Portland Place
London W1B 1LY
Helpline. 020 7436 5881
www.uk-sands.org

Twin Research Unit
St Thomas' Hospital
Block 4A
1st Floor
South Wing
London SE1 7EH
www.twin-research.ac.uk

UK Twin to Twin Transfusion
Syndrome Association
Tel. 020 8581 7359
www.twin2twin.co.uk

Working Families (information
on childcare and employment
rights)
1–3 Berry Street
London EC1V 0AA
Tel. 020 7253 7243
www.workingfamilies.org.uk

Other Resources

Tamba *Buggy and Pushchair Guide*

An 8 page booklet to help you find the right buggy or pushchair for your multiples. Only £2.50 including p&p. Orders can be taken over the phone using a credit or debit card on 0870 770 3305.

Triplet and Quad Pushchairs

Lotsofbabies Ltd
58 Cavendish Road
Salford
Greater Manchester M7 4NQ
Tel. 0161 740 9979
www.lotsofbabies.com

Two, Four, Six, Eight

A website set up by David Hay and Pat Preedy on educating twins, triplets and more
www.twinsandmultiples.org

INDEX